TABLE OF CONTI

Foreword 3

About the Author 4

Don't Let the Coroner be the First to Identify Your Disease 5

The Biggest & Worst Pandemic? 8

What is Atherosclerosis? 11

What is Chronic Disease and Can it be Cured? 14

What is Cardiometabolic Disease? 16

Stroke or Heart Attack: What Really Happens? 17

Red Flags for Arterial & Other Chronic Diseases 18

What is Insulin Resistance? Can it be Reversed? 19

How Does the CureCenter Measure Arterial Disease and Root Causes? 24

My Ultrasound Revealed Atherosclerosis. What's Next? 27

My Ultrasound <u>Did Not</u> Reveal Atherosclerosis. What Now? 29

What is a Coronary Artery Calcium Score? 30

What is a Carotid Intima Media Thickness (CIMT) Ultrasound? 32

Life Line Screening 35

You Have the Power: Improve Your Health 36

What Will My Providers Say About My CurePlan? 37

How Do I Optimize My Diet for Prevention of Chronic Disease? 39

What Foods Should I Eat and What Should I Avoid? 41

What Are Healthy Ways to Cook? 44

How Can I Use CureCoach.App to Measure My Nutrition? 46

What is Body Composition Analysis? 47

What is Visceral Fat & How Do I Reduce it? 48

What is Continuous Glucose Monitoring (CGM)? 51

What is the Difference Between a CurePlan and the Ornish Reversal Program? 52

How Does Vitamin D Deficiency Affect My Health? 54

Are Supplements Beneficial? 57

Statins: The Rest of the Story 60

Why is Oral Health Important to My Overall Health? 66

How Can My Oral Health Professionals Support My Optimal Health? .. 69

What is Sleep Apnea? Why Should I Test for it? 74

What is Lipoprotein A/Lp(a)? Does it Increase risk for Heart Attack & Stroke? 76

What Are LDL and HDL? How Do They Affect My Health? 78

Genetic Testing: How Does it Impact Arterial Disease? 80

Covid-19: What Should I Know? What Should I Do? 85

Conclusion 88

FOREWORD

It is a profound honor to contribute this foreword to CURE, a publication that reflects both the depth and breadth of Dr. Craig Backs' commitment to transforming how we approach chronic disease. Having had the privilege of attending the BaleDoneen preceptorship alongside Dr. Backs over a decade ago, I witnessed firsthand his dedication to exploring innovative, evidence-based preventive strategies in medicine. What began as a shared journey to better understand the intricate connections between oral and systemic health has, for both of us, evolved into a mission to reshape the very foundation of healthcare.

In dentistry, my professional pivot led to the creation of the Larkin Protocol and Proactive Oral Wellness, where I've focused on integrating advanced salivary diagnostics, periodontal therapy, and systemic health screening into routine dental care. Dr. Backs, in parallel, has spearheaded groundbreaking initiatives at The CureCenter for Chronic Disease, where he has redefined how we prevent, manage, and even reverse chronic conditions. Both of us have witnessed the power of early detection and prevention in improving patient outcomes—and more importantly, in saving lives.

CURE represents more than a publication; it is a manifesto for the future of healthcare. Dr. Backs masterfully illuminates the path forward, demonstrating how personalized, preventive protocols can disrupt the cycle of chronic disease and restore hope to patients and providers alike. His insights are a call to action for practitioners across disciplines to adopt a more integrative and patient-centered approach.

Our shared history with the BaleDoneen Method underscored an enduring truth: the interconnectivity of the human body demands collaboration between disciplines. Dr. Backs exemplifies this principle, building bridges between medicine, dentistry, and beyond to address the root causes of illness rather than merely its symptoms.

As you embark on the pages of CURE, prepare to be inspired, challenged, and equipped with tools to transform your understanding of chronic disease prevention. Dr. Backs' work reminds us that true healthcare is proactive, integrative, and deeply personal—a vision I wholeheartedly share.

With admiration and respect,

Thomas Larkin, DDS
Founder, Proactive Oral Wellness | Creator, The Larkin Protocol

ABOUT THE AUTHOR

Craig Backs, MD, is an experienced specialist in Internal Medicine, caring for adults through diagnostic skills and management of acute and chronic disease. These diseases include diabetes, hypertension, atherosclerosis, and other conditions that respond to better lifestyle choices, supplements and medications. Left to progress, they can dramatically shorten or ruin an individual's life. He is best described as an "open minded allopath" now focused on root cause elimination, correction of nutrient deficiencies with targeted supplements and medication when the benefit outweighs the risk.

Dr. Backs was educated at Valparaiso University and Southern Illinois University School of Medicine. His Internal Medicine residency was completed at SIU School of Medicine in Springfield, IL. It was there he practiced with a group of other internists and primary care doctors. He served as President of the Illinois State Medical Society among other leadership roles. After three years as Chief Medical Officer at St. John's Hospital in Springfield, IL, he opened The Center for Prevention Heart Attack and Stroke, which later became The CureCenter for Chronic Disease. Dr. Backs has made it his mission to cure Chronic Disease by digging out its root causes.

His personal journey to cure Chronic Disease began in May of 2012. "My own personal health went through a dramatic makeover," says Dr. Backs. "I now know better and provide a more credible example for my patients. I understand the challenges they face as they pursue a healthier lifestyle. I know how to motivate and coach success."

Dr. Backs uses his personal and professional experience to develop and coach your Personalized CurePlan to prevent and reverse chronic disease into remission and live a long optimally healthy life.

Learn more about the personal health journey of Dr. Craig Backs by scanning the QR code.

DON'T LET THE CORONER BE THE FIRST TO IDENTIFY YOUR DISEASE

I once met with a man in his 60's who I cared for years ago. He was interested in reconnecting because his current physician had retired. After speaking with him, I offered to develop a custom CurePlan (the personalized plans I offer my patients to help them gain optimal health). He declined and stated, "I eat right, I exercise, and my doctor says my cholesterol is good." I decided to not push the issue because it rarely, if ever, works to change beliefs.

A few weeks later, I received a call from the hospital. It was this man's wife, informing me that he had suffered cardiac arrest while exercising the prior morning. He had been successfully resuscitated and was recovering without apparent residual effects. He now wanted to discuss a CurePlan because his catheterization had demonstrated three vessel coronary artery disease and he was recommended for coronary bypass surgery. He asked: "What should I do?"

Sadly, I had little to offer and urged him to follow the advice he had received for standard care. I had no influence on his hospital care other than as a "friend." I wanted to avoid creating friction with his surgeon and other doctors.

I could have suggested he go home, visit me to discuss the details, and then decide if surgery, with all its risks, was the correct option. However, I did not believe it was worth the risk of him going into cardiac arrest again outside of the hospital. I also didn't have all of the details of his diagnosis and he had previously declined my offer for a custom CurePlan and advice for proactive measures.

So, he and his family experienced a life-altering operation on the heels of a life-altering cardiac arrest and resuscitation. All of this would likely have been avoided if he had known of his arterial disease early and proactively treated the missed root causes.

I hope that anyone who reads this story will be proactive in their own interest and for the benefit of their loved ones. It is crucial to identify the disease that lurks within and could turn fatal without warning.

You are at higher risk of a stroke or heart attack than you think. Atherosclerosis is the highest cause of death and disability in countries around the world, including the United States. The risk is more significant than all types of cancer combined.

Most of the time, the first symptom is a disabling stroke or a lethal heart attack. The very words "stroke" and "heart attack" convey the sudden and serious events requiring rapid rescue. When seconds count, you'll be waiting several minutes for the ambulance to arrive. In fact, 90 minutes is considered a good standard time for opening clogged arteries; and that is if you are able to get to a tertiary medical center with an interventional cardiologist on call.

There is a solution - an opportunity for durable remission - a CURE. Take proactive, affordable steps to see into your future and improve it. It is not as hard or expensive as you have been led to believe. In fact, it is far more possible than the Standard American Doctor (SAD) knows or would be allowed to deliver.

What we'll cover:

This booklet will get to the point, provide clear and concise information, and introduce you to The CureCenter for Chronic Disease and your personal CurePlan. Get started on your own proactive path to remission from the silent killer that can be stopped long before it becomes a threat.

There are many "wellness" programs and initiatives. Prevention is clearly the optimal approach to any problem. But, in reality, most of us are well beyond the opportunity for prevention of progressive atherosclerosis/arterial disease. I believe we need proactive, systemic, and holistic lifestyle and medical intervention to preempt the need for rescue/procedural interventions for unplanned events.

Many approach this in other ways, expecting you to spend time and monetize their books, podcasts/social media and proprietary supplements. If you are looking for a lot of detail and long conversations intended to prove expertise, I'm not your guy. I've been told I have a face for radio and a voice for print.

I prefer accomplishment over activity, results over talk, and efficient use of time, testing, and money.

Read on to learn about our CurePlan process that has protected thousands from suffering a stroke or heart attack since 2015.

When I first encountered the Bale Doneen Method and its guarantee of results, I was skeptical. However, after a decade of not losing a single patient to a heart attack or stroke, I'm glad I shifted course to provide this opportunity to my patients. You deserve better than what is offered by the health care system.

My mission is to make the highly effective and proactive principles of the Bale Doneen Method and other programs affordable and accessible for everyone who needs them. My goal is to focus on what is most effective and use digital tools to communicate and deliver the best individualized, evidence-based care. Don't waste time and money to support ineffective systems and bureaucracies.

Read on. Open your mind to the possibility of a CURE for your chronic arterial and metabolic disease. When you are ready to move forward with your own CurePlan, schedule a Discovery Zoom Call at theCureCenter.life/discovery-call.

Craig Backs MD

THE BIGGEST & WORST PANDEMIC?

There is a **CURE**. We can stop the **C**atastrophic **U**nseen **R**eversible **E**pidemic of Cardiometabolic Disease.

Arterial/cardiometabolic disease is the chronic condition with acute manifestations most responsible for destroying our population. It continues to shorten and ruin more lives than COVID and all cancers combined.

The disease starts (earlier than we'd like to think) as arterial injury leading to inflammation and plaque formation. We often first take notice when it becomes symptomatic in the form of a stroke, heart attack, dementia, kidney disease, or peripheral vascular disease. **It is preventable, reversible and Curable in the sense of long-term, stable remission.**

Forty years of practicing medicine has taught me that most of us are **NOT** motivated to change or become more healthy. This is especially true when we are addicted to toxic food and behaviors that are highly promoted and subsidized by cultural propaganda and public policy. Public health recommendations are making the problem worse, not better, by incompetence and corrupting industry influence.

Pain, suffering, and fear of loss tend to be the urgent factors that motivate us to seek help and make sacrifices, giving up the "good" for something better. These same factors lead us to purchase life and disability insurance. I believe we should instead invest in health assurance.

While prevention is the best approach to any problem, **most of us are past the point where prevention is possible**. We need to see it, measure it, and stop progression to achieve/sustain remission. We need to heal the injury for a long-term CURE, both individually and as communities.

Additionally, the contribution of oral inflammation (infected teeth/inflamed gums) is almost universally overlooked. Dental professionals have the opportunity to offer an alternative when working in collaboration with proactive medical professionals who look beyond the traditional risk factors of hyperlipidemia, smoking and hypertension. These include insulin resistance (a feature, not a bug, for our hunter/gatherer optimization), exposure to oxidative stress from the environment, vitamin D deficiency, homocysteine elevation, lipoprotein(a) and others.

This type of CURE should be available to anyone, regardless of their financial status. Success often does not come from a radical change in behavior. Instead, it comes from a series of nudges that are reinforced by seeing measurable progress in areas such as:

- **Body Composition:** measures of insulin resistance: Visceral/% Body Fat
- **Blood test indicators of inflammation:** hsCRP, LpPLA2, Microalbumin/Creatinine ratio
- **Ultrasound** measured arterial intima media thickness/age/inflammation

A case study to consider:

Recently, I performed carotid ultrasound scans and body composition analyses on 39 employees of a rural business.

The CEO, a patient in my proactive medicine practice, leads by example. He made an investment in his employees to offer the opportunity to see their individual threats (arterial plaque and inflammation) and pursue the opportunity to heal. He also provided them with free access to vitamin D, vitamin C, zinc, and other supplements and allowed each employee to decide whether they would benefit from COVID mRNA injections.

These were hard working, skilled, blue collar, agricultural workers with lower-than-average access to mainstream healthcare. Their age range was 18-79 and job descriptions ranged from CEO to janitor.

With the support of resources such as our secure, digital platform, CureCoach. app, reports were sent to employees within one day.

The findings were typical of the population at large:

- 23 of the 39 (59%) had visible arterial injury that can be healed, postponing indefinitely disabling strokes and life-ending/changing heart attacks, rehabilitation, stents or bypass surgery.
- 20 of the 37 (54%) had a visceral fat level consistent with inflammatory insulin resistance. This is the most prevalent driver of chronic inflammation and progresses to prediabetes and Type 2 Diabetes.

Those with detected arterial injury or elevated levels of visceral fat were offered a 30 minute Discovery Zoom Call to review reports and discuss next steps.

I'm pleased to report that many have taken advantage of these Discovery Zoom Calls and most are pursuing further lab assessment and consultation.

Lessons learned:

- We TALK about prevention but we ACT to intervene when motivated by pain, suffering or visible/palpable evidence of injury or illness.
- We need less talk and more action. Scan and measure first. Address questions later. Replace the risk model with a measurable disease model.

- Risk calculation is replaced by disease revelation, measurement and monitoring of the changes from intervention. A proactive lifestyle and medical intervention strategy outperforms a prevention or intervention strategy for those already afflicted by silent but deadly progressive arterial injury.
- A small efficient team with digital, cloud-based tools can accomplish more at a lower cost (time and treasure) than the current bloated reactive system. That system depends on chronic disease and its complications for revenue to support bloated facilities, teams, and bureaucracies that have nothing to do with care and everything to do with optimizing profit margins.
- The key to success is motivation provoked by awareness, concern, open mindedness, and coachability. Not education, wealth, or social status.
- A picture is worth a thousand words. A video is worth far more. Personally seeing ultrasound images of arterial injury with an opportunity to heal it motivates change. This is what we offer at the CureCenter. Simply seeing reduces risk for heart attack and stroke by 50% in just one year.
- Population improvement can begin organically, one individual at a time, then at scale.
- We should not wait for the government or other authorities to act. They won't change themselves and we don't have the time. People are needlessly suffering and dying for lack of access to optimal, achievable remedies and results.
- Focus on arterial injury (Inflammation and plaque) and reduction of visceral fat (insulin resistance). This focus is achievable and improves general wellness by measuring reliable indicators of chronic inflammation due to oxidative stress.
- Rural and blue collar workers deserve this opportunity as much as urban executives and the laptop class. They are just as likely (or perhaps even more likely) to succeed with the right kind of coaching. I believe this is because they are less controlled by the current mainstream health care processes and incentives.

This case study is just the start. Our process is scalable, effective and far more affordable than alternatives.

After seeing 1,000+ patients over the past decade, not a single patient who followed our CurePlan has suffered a stroke or heart attack. This is dramatic evidence of efficacy and a huge threat to the medical industrial pharma payer business model.

WHAT IS ATHEROSCLEROSIS?

Atherosclerosis is injury and inflammation of the artery wall. Healthy arteries are important because they carry oxygen-rich blood from the heart to the entire body's tissue and organs. A more accurate description of the most dangerous stage of disease would be "**artheritis**" or "**arthritis**" meaning inflammation of the arteries. "**Sclerosis**" or hardening/calcification is a later healed more benign stage of the disease.

Acne is a relevant analogy most of us know. Inflammation in the skin (artery wall) creates pimples/plaque (in areas where turbulence adds mechanical shearing forces) that are prone to rupture (homogeneous and heterogeneous plaque) when new. The preferred path is to heal and leave a scar. When plaque is becoming calcified, it is healing. Rising coronary calcium score is a good, not bad, trend if you are on a healing program.

Atherosclerosis is often called "hardening of the arteries" due to a buildup of calcium deposits in plaque that forms in the arteries. However, **calcium presence is actually a sign of healing** and increases over time with new plaque development (bad) and current plaque calcifying (good). Plaque that has little or no fibrosis or calcium is less stable, more prone to rupture, and more threatening.

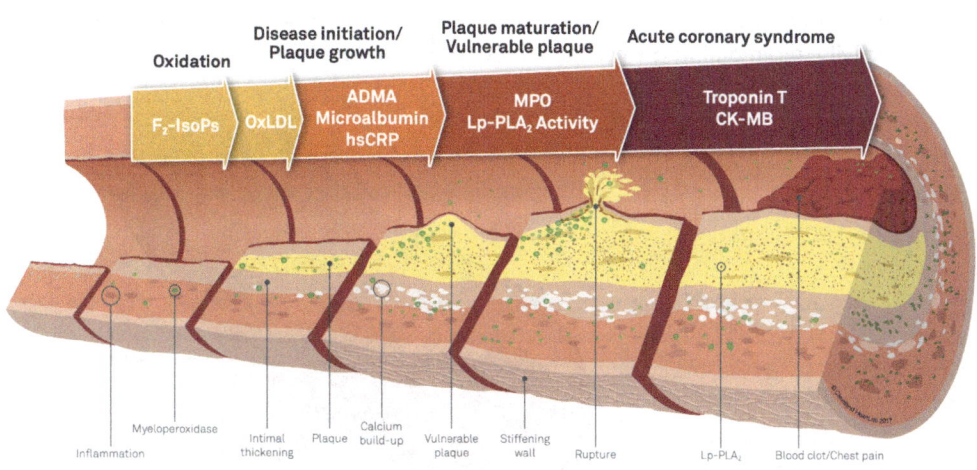

Image Source: Cleveland Heart Lab

When your artery walls thicken with plaque and narrow the lumen, blood flow to any organ can be reduced or interrupted, leading to disability (temporary or permanent) or death. Stress tests and angiograms are useful to detect this phenomenon. However, the greatest danger is sudden plaque rupture and blood clot formation, resulting in heart attack or stroke. The best test to evaluate this stage is ultrasound for the carotid arteries (affordable) and AI processed coronary artery CT (expensive).

The heart pumps blood into the aorta and arteries, which then branch out into smaller blood vessels, eventually delivering the oxygen and nutrients to individual cells. Without healthy arteries, the body's tissues and organs would not receive the oxygen and nutrients needed to function properly. Maintaining healthy arteries is crucial for overall health and wellbeing.

Arterial health improvement is a great reflection of reduced oxidative stress, inflammation and overall health improvement.

The artery wall has three layers:

- **Adventitia** (outer layer): composed of connective tissue that supports and protects the artery from external injury.
- **Media** (middle layer): made of smooth muscle and elastic fibers. It is responsible for regulating the diameter of the artery, which affects blood pressure and blood flow.
- **Intima** (inner layer): a thin layer of endothelial cells that regulate all kinds of activity, maintaining a smooth surface for blood to flow through.

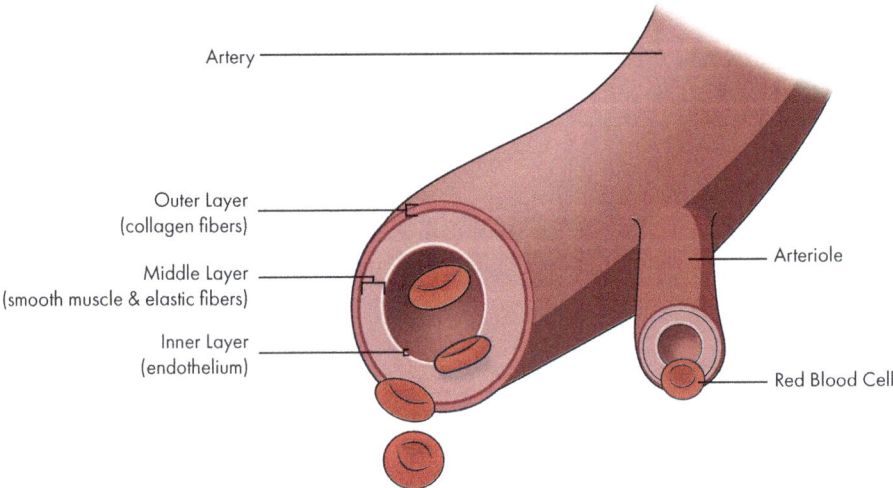

Image Source: NIH U.S. National Library of Medicine

What causes plaque to develop in the arteries?

Plaque grows due to complicated interactions between genetics, high blood pressure, lipids, inflammation driven by oxidative stress and insulin resistance, diabetes, and other conditions. Arterial disease is like acne and plaque is like a pimple or pustule.

Plaque progresses as follows:

- **Homogeneous plaque**: This fresh, soft vulnerable plaque is like a new pimple. It is the most dangerous stage of plaque evolution because it is most likely to rupture and cause a heart attack or stroke.
- **Heterogeneous plaque**: This type of plaque is like a pimple that is healing. It can still rupture or erode because inflammation has not resolved. It is the most common stage of plaque seen on imaging of arteries. It is an uneven buildup of inflammatory material, fibrin, and calcium.
- **Calcified Plaque**: This type of plaque is the scar that results when plaque heals. Like any scar, we carry it for the rest of our lives but we carry it for the rest of our lives but it is no longer a threat. Calcified plaque is the residual scar of a rupture-related event that could have happened, but didn't! Calcified plaque is less likely to rupture, but can still cause problems by narrowing the artery and restricting blood flow.

As plaque is developing, it is vulnerable to rupture. A clot forms in the artery lumen. If the clot blocks an artery feeding your heart, you experience a heart attack. If it blocks an artery feeding your brain, you experience a stroke. Both can result in death or disability, but they can also be prevented by making artery walls thinner/less inflamed and healthier.

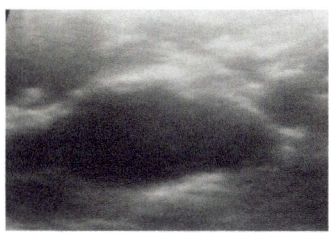 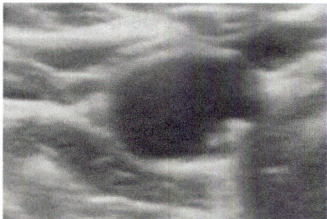

No Plaque **Heterogeneous Plaque**

Atherosclerosis and its progression is more common but not inevitable as we age. Most adults have it starting in the thirties.

Using new science, testing, and treatments, we can halt and reverse the disease in our arteries.

WHAT IS CHRONIC DISEASE AND CAN IT BE CURED?

A chronic disease is a medical condition that persists over a long period of time, typically for years. Chronic diseases can significantly impact your quality of life. Examples include diabetes, hypertension, atherosclerosis (arterial disease), dementia, and certain types of cancer. Chronic diseases are caused by an interaction of genetic, environmental, and lifestyle factors. They become more common as we age.

The chronic diseases listed above (among others) are co-morbid, which means more than one typically coexist in the same individual. They interact to cause harm. The root causes include a refined, processed, carbohydrate-rich diet, sedentary lifestyle, high levels of stress, sleep disturbances, and smoking interacting with genetic tendencies.

At the CureCenter, we emphasize the bad S's: Sweets, Starches, Snacks, Seed oils, Sitting Salt, Smoking, Sleep/Snoring disorders, Stress and Sexual Starvation. We promote a diet of real unprocessed food and exercise, augmented with supplements and medications for specific needs. But at least stop eating processed food, sweats and starches.

Why is it important to reverse chronic disease into remission or cure?

Events such as heart attack and stroke can become lethal quickly. However, they are actually caused by years of silent, unknown chronic disease which progresses to atherosclerosis/arterial disease. Plaque rupture or erosion is the first step in the cascade leading to the blood clots that suddenly interrupt blood flow. Changing your lifestyle and reversing chronic disease is not just important for your overall general health. It significantly reduces your risk of serious, disabling and fatal events such as heart attack or stroke.

Reversal of chronic disease will also improve overall quality of life by reducing common symptoms such as fatigue or difficulty breathing. It can prevent further complications and development of other serious diseases.

Why have I been told that chronic disease is manageable, but not reversible?

Let's be honest. The business of mainstream medical care is Chronic Disease Management. Mainstream medicine is simply overseeing our health decline with "management" of chronic disease. It sets you up to be vulnerable to inevitable exposure to Covid, flu, and other external threats. We can do better.

The "Standard of Care" goal is to manage the disease and treat its complications. Costly and profitable drugs and procedures are the mainstay of treatment with this plan, with costs rapidly rising to unsustainable levels. We may live longer, but we're sick and racking up costs and treatments. Keep in mind: Your costs are revenue for the medical system, including health insurance.

You are not the customer. You are the product.

Good News: Chronic disease can be prevented, reversed, put into remission, and even Cured!

It is reversed by better choices about nutrition and activity interacting with our genes and environment. Quit smoking, avoid alcohol and drug abuse, avoid sugar and processed foods (sweets, starches, and snacks) and get off the couch. Be aware of the addictive nature of processed foods and find support to overcome craving for them.

Our mission is to discover and measure your chronic disease, identify your individual root causes, develop a Personalized CurePlan to reverse it, and demonstrate measurable improvement.

When improvement or remission lasts long enough, it's reasonable to call it "cured." No cure is 100% effective or lasts forever, but this cure can endure for years if we do the right things.

At the CureCenter, we Measure, Motivate, Mentor, Measure again, and Maintain Momentum. We call these our healthy M&M's! They are good for you and can cure your chronic disease by restoring your health.

Here is a fun and handy acronym to summarize: SAM

S's - Sweets, Starches, Snacks, Seed oils, Sitting, Stress, (poor) Sleep/Snoring, Salt, Smoking & Sexual Starvation.

Causes:

A's (Added) - Arterial disease, Diabetes, Dementia, Erectile dysfunction, Depression

Cured by:

M's - Measure, Motivate, Mentor, Monitor, Maintain Momentum

WHAT IS CARDIOMETABOLIC DISEASE?

Cardiometabolic disease, also known as atherosclerosis (arterial disease) dyslipidemia and metabolic syndrome, refers to a cluster of conditions that increase the risk of developing cardiovascular diseases and type 2 diabetes. It is caused by a combination of factors that affect metabolism, chronic inflammation and the cardiovascular system. These include obesity, high blood pressure (hypertension), hyperinsulinemia (insulin resistance or diabetes), and high oxidized LDL cholesterol and triglyceride levels.

The exact cause of cardiometabolic disease is not fully understood. It is likely a result of a combination of genetic factors, adverse lifestyle choices, and environmental toxins that create oxidative stress. Sedentary lifestyle, unhealthy diet (processed foods, starch and sugars), smoking, excessive alcohol consumption, and chronic stress are among the contributing factors.

When you have cardiometabolic disease, you are at a higher risk of developing serious health complications, such as heart disease, stroke, and diabetes. These conditions can lead to significant disability and mortality rates if not identified and proactively treated.

The diagnosis of cardiometabolic disease is typically based on the presence of specific risk criteria, including abdominal obesity (measured by body composition or waist circumference), elevated blood pressure, high blood sugar levels, elevated oxidized LDL and triglycerides, and low levels of high-density lipoprotein (HDL) cholesterol.

Reversal of cardiometabolic disease includes lifestyle modifications, such as adopting a low carb diet, regular physical activity, weight loss, and smoking cessation. Medications may also be prescribed to control blood pressure, blood sugar levels, oxidized LDL cholesterol and, most importantly, **inflammation**. Supplements are recommended to treat identified deficiencies like vitamin D and folic acid to reduce homocysteine.

Preventing and reversing cardiometabolic disease requires a comprehensive approach that addresses the underlying risk factors. Promote a healthy lifestyle, educate individuals about the risks associated with cardiometabolic disease, and provide appropriate medical interventions to reduce the impact of this condition on individuals' health and well-being by putting it into remission.

STROKE OR HEART ATTACK: WHAT REALLY HAPPENS?

There are four phases of arterial health:

- Normal Artery
- Vulnerable/Unstable Homogeneous Plaque
- Stable (Fibrous) Heterogeneous Plaque
- Healed Calcified Plaque

A **normal artery** refers to the stage before atherosclerotic plaque forms in the artery wall. This stage is typical of younger individuals. Atherosclerosis is more common with age, but it is not normal "aging."

Stable calcified plaque is like a scar that forms after an injury. It is the latest and most stable stage of the process. It won't disappear altogether, but it also won't cause sudden harm. Calcified and fibrotic connective tissue wall off the plaque from the lumen of the artery where the blood flows. This is like a healed scar from a prior injury, an event that could have but did not happen. The lumen through which blood flows is diminished in size, but the situation is stable. However, it reveals increased risk of forming more plaque in the future because it has done so in the past, especially if the root causes are still active.

Vulnerable/unstable homogeneous new plaque is the real danger. It is actually newly-formed plaque. When plaque forms due to inflammation or injury to the artery wall, there are two potential outcomes: (1) it can heal without causing harm, becoming stable plaque, or (2) it can rupture or erode and trigger formation of a blood clot in the lumen. This blocks blood flow through the artery. That flow interruption kills heart muscle or brain tissue.

Arterial disease is silent, deadly, progressive but preventable and reversible. At the CureCenter, we work with our patients to **prevent the formation of new plaque and heal plaque that has already formed**. We identify and minimize the common and uncommon root causes with a Personalized CurePlan based on better choices, targeted supplements, safe and effective medications and genetic tests that determine individualized therapy.

Are your arteries healthy? If they are sicker and older than you believe, we can make them healthier and younger again.

RED FLAGS FOR ARTERIAL & OTHER CHRONIC DISEASES

There are many conditions associated with arterial and other chronic diseases that lurk silently only to become suddenly lethal. These "red flags" reveal increased risk of heart attack, stroke, and other consequences of chronic disease. They are not clearly causative or modifiable, but they can motivate curiosity.

Pay attention to them. The more red flags you recognize, the more you should want to know what may be lurking in you that could suddenly or slowly cost you your health... or even your life.

In addition to the following red flags, keep in mind that men over 40 years of age, women over 50, and individuals of African-American or Hispanic descent are also at higher risk of chronic disease.

Risk factors include:

- Personal or family history of cardiovascular/arterial disease, heart attack, stroke, or Type 2 Diabetes
- Age: men over 40 and women over 50
- Gestational diabetes
- Elevated cholesterol
- Nicotine use in any form (including second-hand smoke)
- Psychosocial issues such as depression, anxiety, or stress
- High blood pressure
- Abdominal obesity (high levels of visceral fat)
- Sleep problems (not enough sleep, sleep apnea, etc.)
- Periodontal/Endodontal disease
- Erectile dysfunction
- Rheumatoid arthritis
- Lupus
- Psoriasis
- Migraine headaches
- Gout
- Polycystic ovaries
- Hirsutism (facial hair growth in women)
- Osteoporosis
- Pre-eclampsia
- Breast cancer treatment
- COVID spike protein infection or injection

WHAT IS INSULIN RESISTANCE? CAN IT BE REVERSED?

Insulin resistance occurs when the cells of the muscles, fat, and liver become insensitive or resistant to insulin, causing the body to produce higher insulin levels to compensate. This state of **hyperinsulinemia** is highly inflammatory for your entire body, especially your arteries and nerves. Eventually insulin production fails and blood sugar levels begin to rise. It is at this point the patient is diagnosed with diabetes based on elevated blood glucose/"sugar", the final stage of "diabesity."

However, even thin, lean people can be insulin resistant, especially if muscle mass is low (sarcopenia) relative to body fat, especially visceral fat.

In reality, **insulin resistance is so common that we should assume its presence until proven absent.** Why is it so common to be called a "feature" rather than a "bug"? Why wouldn't evolutionary pressures get rid of it? The answer: It is an adaptation to the hunter gatherer lifestyle. It is not well suited for our current cultural promotion of "grazing" constantly on sweets, starches and highly processed snacking. And, it doesn't cause death prior to reproduction.

The answer: **Eat like a hunter gatherer!** Eat within a short time window (six hours is ideal) and eat lots of vegetables, some fruit (sugary!), meat/protein and good fat (olive, coconut or avocado oil, seeds, nuts).

What is Diabesity?

Diabesity is the spectrum of adverse health effects of diabetes and obesity. It is the result of a modern environment of processed food loaded with sweets and starches consumed throughout the day.

Before rising glucose levels are detected, the higher insulin levels (caused by insulin resistance) raise blood pressure and create inflammation that contributes to arterial damage. We call this damage atherosclerosis. It can also lead to diabetes, dementia (Type 3 Diabetes?), erectile dysfunction, and depression. Risk of heart attack, stroke, and dementia also increase.

We develop "tolerance" to the toxic effects of sweets and insulin. This leads us to crave more sweets, driving our insulin levels higher, and can lead to early death and disability if unrecognized and untreated.

This graph illustrates the relationship between insulin resistance, rising insulin levels, and blood glucose levels associated with the progression from prediabetes to Type 2 Diabetes. It should be labeled "The Natural History of "Diabesity."

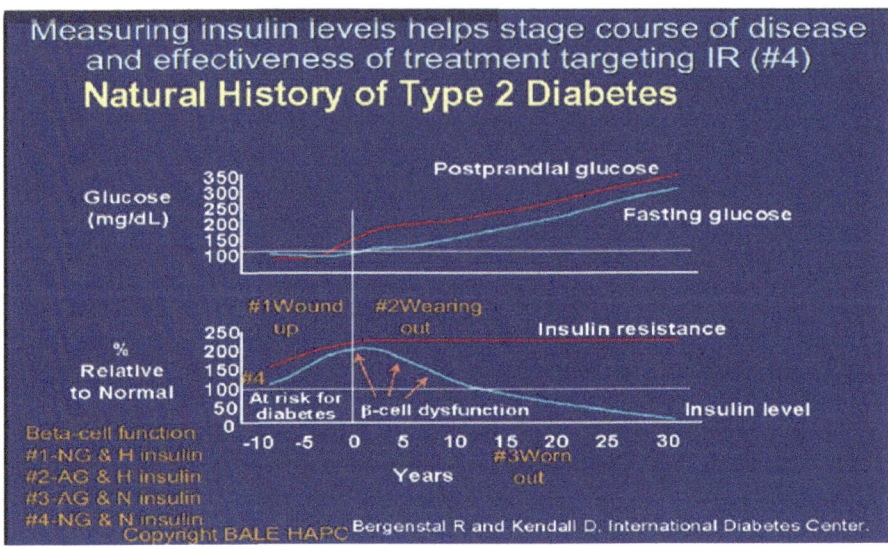

Image Source: International Diabetes Center

What are some indicators of Insulin Resistance/Diabesity?

Some indicators of insulin resistance include (but are not limited to):

- Increased waist size
- Elevated visceral fat
- High blood pressure
- Elevated blood sugar
- High triglycerides
- Low HDL cholesterol (Metabolic syndrome)
- Small dense LDL predominance (Pattern B)
- Heart attack or stroke
- Gestational diabetes
- Polycystic Ovary Syndrome
- Erectile Dysfunction
- Ananthosis Nigricans
- Periodontal disease

How do we identify Insulin Resistance/Diabesity?

The gold standard identifier of insulin resistance includes a two hour oral glucose tolerance test with simultaneous insulin levels. During this test, your blood is drawn before and after drinking a sugary liquid to see how your body responds. Measuring against certain high benchmarks define diabetes and prediabetes. Normal glucose (blood sugar) levels should be below 125 after one hour of this test and 120 after two hours.

Fasting glucose levels above 90 should raise concerns about insulin resistance until other measures are used to rule it out.

Other measures used to identify insulin resistance include: high triglycerides, low high-density lipoprotein (HDL), small and dense low-density lipoprotein (LDL), hypertension, non-alcoholic fatty liver disease (NAFLD), and idiopathic neuropathy.

At the CureCenter, we perform body composition analyses on all of our patients to help identify insulin resistance/diabesity. Elevated visceral fat (which correlates with percent body fat) can be detected in a few minutes, revealing some of the earliest evidence.

Visceral fat can be hard to identify without a body composition analysis, as one may appear "thin" on the outside, but still have high levels of visceral fat. These healthy looking individuals have low muscle mass, known as sarcopenia. This occurs most commonly in women after they experience menopause, especially if they avoid resistance exercises.

How do we reverse Insulin Resistance/Diabesity?

- **Dietary Changes**: First, cut out sweets, starches, and snacks from your diet. Excess sugar in your daily diet is stored as fat, worsening insulin resistance. Avoid sugar, artificial sweeteners (gateway drugs that also increase insulin levels), processed foods, and white bread, pasta, potatoes, and rice. These all raise insulin levels (even in the absence of high amounts of calories) and perpetuate cravings for sweets. These cravings can lead to food addiction, much like addictions to drugs and alcohol.

  In order to effectively reverse insulin resistance/diabesity, be sure to eat more vegetables, protein, and good fats (from sources such as nuts, seeds, and fish. Fruit contains vitamins as well as toxic sugar. Eat it in moderation

  Fruit is higher in sugar if dried or juiced. Eat whole fruit in limited amounts. Berries are the best. Bananas and grapes are like candy bars and M&Ms!

- **Exercise**: Get off the couch. A sedentary lifestyle is a recipe for all types of chronic disease. While nearly all types of physical activity can be beneficial, we recommend high intensity interval training and building muscle through resistance training in addition to aerobic/cardio exercise.

- **Time Restricted (Window) Feeding/Fasting**: At the CureCenter, we see the best results in individuals who restrict their good food intake to an 8-hour window each day. In the other 16 hours of the day, drink only water or unsweetened beverages.

For additional information about healthy fasting, we recommend resources created by Dr. Jason Fung, including his books, "The Obesity Code," and "The Diabetes Code," blog (The Fasting Method), and YouTube channel.

- **Proper Amounts of Sleep**: Poor amount and quality of sleep has been linked to higher levels of insulin resistance. Be sure to get proper amounts of sleep each night. More is generally better. Very few of us get enough sleep. It is rare to get too much sleep.

- **Manage Stress**: High levels of stress have been linked to insulin resistance. Although it's not always easy, try to find ways to relieve stress to reduce cortisol levels that can raise glucose and insulin.

  Exercise is a proven and healthy way to reduce stress, so get off the couch and go outdoors or to the gym. Mindfulness practices such as meditation, prayer, or yoga can also help to manage stress.

- **Measure Your Results**: When you first start on your journey to reverse resistance to insulin, it's best to measure your results every 1-2 weeks by taking a body composition test (these can be done at the CureCenter office). When you've met your goal, continue to test every 1-2 months to ensure you are staying on track. Staying accountable is key. Seeing improvement perpetuates the process.

  We call it M&M's (the healthy kind): Measure, Motivate, and Maintain Momentum.

- **Supplements and Medication (if goals not achieved by lifestyle changes alone)**: Sometimes, insulin resistance is so stubborn that a healthy diet and exercise do not achieve the desired reduction in fat. This can be due to an incomplete commitment to carbohydrate restriction or insufficient patience. We cannot out-prescribe a bad diet. However, sometimes a little help is needed. At the CureCenter, we will prescribe medications and/or supplements that best suit your needs and lifestyle.

  I'm often asked about metformin. Metformin reduces glucose primarily by reducing release of glucose from liver stores of glycogen, but it is also considered an insulin sensitizer. There is a lot of interest in it as an anti-aging and anticancer treatment. Its impact on cardiovascular outcomes is not as impressive as pioglitazone, a thiazolidinedione medication.

- **Pioglitazone** improves insulin sensitivity. It is generic and has been around for a long time. It suffers from a bad reputation for fluid retention because its use has been delayed till patients with Type 2 Diabetes fail 1st line drugs that increase the risk of heart damage from heart attacks and restricted blood flow. But when used in the prediabetes stage, before damage to the heart, it is well tolerated. It dramatically reduces the risk of heart attack (>70% reduction) while lowering insulin levels.

HOW DOES THE CURECENTER MEASURE ARTERIAL DISEASE AND ROOT CAUSES?

The inflammation nature of arterial disease (which causes heart attack, stroke and dementia) is not the basis of mainstream medical care. New testing methods and technology enable the CureCenter to offer more individualized and effective treatments.

We perform these tests that are not generally available from standard care. While there are threshold values that define categories, **the key is to promote favorable trends**, even when good. The goal is **better** on our way to **optimal**:

- **Carotid Intima Media Thickness (CIMT) Testing**: CIMT measures arterial wall thickness/sickness/inflammation. It documents atherosclerotic plaque stage and nature. A thicker artery wall is an inflamed, older and sicker artery wall. This indicator of arterial inflammation predicts formation of atherosclerotic plaque and related events such as heart attack and stroke.

  Arterial wall thickness (inflammation) is more relevant than luminal "blockage" in predicting new and unstable plaque formation. Unstable plaque rupture is the event experienced as a heart attack or stroke. This is more likely with new homogeneous unstable plaque. It becomes less likely as plaque becomes more homogeneous/healing and is minimal when plaque is calcified/healed/stable. Proactive optimal care can heal arterial disease and make your arteries healthier and younger with less risk of disability, death or need for rescue intervention procedures.

- **Screening carotid ultrasound (CureScreen)**: This limited lower cost carotid ultrasound (using point of care Butterfly iQ probe) is like a screening pap smear, mammogram or PSA to detect early cancer. If we find no disease, peace of mind is the benefit. If, however, even a little bit of arterial disease is found (like a little bit of cancer) the images can be sent for a CIMT report (see above) and then compared over time to make sure you are safer by following your CurePlan.

- **LpPLA2 (PLAC) Test**: This enzyme rises when plaque and artery walls are inflamed or "hot." You want your artery wall to be "cool." LpPLA2 drops with a less inflammatory diet, exercise, reduced insulin resistance, supplements (niacin, and bergamot) and statins. It is a fire alarm or "meat thermometer" for arterial wall inflammation.

- **Myeloperoxidase (MPO)**: A rise in MPO should trigger a search for neutrophil involved inflammation, especially from the mouth. MPO indicates inflammation and erosion of the inner lining of the artery known as endothelium. A sudden rise should trigger a search for the inflammation that can cause arterial inflammation, leading to heart attack or stroke. Think of a caustic chemical spill inside your arteries. Like a skin abrasion, blood clots form and can occlude flow.

- **Microalbumin/Creatinine Ratio (MACR)**: MACR rises when blood pressure and blood glucose are poorly controlled. This causes dysfunction of the arterial wall endothelium, allowing albumin to leak into the urine in greater amounts. A leaky endothelium fails to protect the intima from processes that lead to inflammation. Think of it as a smoke detector.

    For more information about these and other tests, visit knowyourrisk.com. You can find additional information from Cleveland Heart Lab, a major source of our testing.

- **Haptoglobin Genotype**: Your Haptoglobin genotype determines if Vitamin E offers protection or increases risk of arterial disease. In addition, individuals with the Hp 1-2 and especially the Hp 2-2 genome are more sensitive to gluten, forming an inflammatory mediator called zonulin that makes your gut "leaky" and raises the risk of autoimmune disease.

- **Insulin Resistance Testing**: Optimally measured through an oral glucose tolerance test, insulin resistance (prediabetes) testing is important in identifying individuals who could be developing vascular complications before a Type 2 Diabetes diagnosis. The glucose tolerance test can identify insulin resistance long before the glucose starts to rise.

    However, if there is other evidence of insulin resistance, we can skip the glucose tolerance test. Clues are seen in levels of HbA1c >5.0, glucose > 90, triglycerides above 100, low HDL, and presence of small dense LDL (Pattern B).

    The earliest detection for insulin resistance can be measured through body composition testing. At the CureCenter, we use the InBody 570, a device that can monitor insulin resistance response to changes in diet. Reducing insulin resistance is generally better for everyone, regardless of risk.

Homocysteine elevation increases risk of:

- Osteoporosis - bone thinning
- Atherosclerosis
- Thrombosis (blood clotting)
- Heart Attack
- Stroke
- Dementia
- Kidney failure
- Neuropathy

Treatment is supplementation with methylated folic acid. Dietary sources of methylated folic acid are leafy greens like spinach and kale.

- **Coronary Artery Calcium Score (CACS):** This CT scan detects mature healed calcified plaque in the coronary arteries. However, it can miss new noncalcified plaque. This test is not useful in monitoring therapy progress/benefit. We recommend CACS when CIMT does not reveal disease but there is still suspicion of coronary artery disease. If this test detects disease that would have otherwise been undetected, a more proactive approach to address root causes will be encouraged. Beware of the slippery slope to a stress test, stents or surgery. Coronary Calcium Score is a "loss leader" for interventional cardiology programs. Call us first before scheduling further tests.

- **Home Sleep Testing and Auto Titrated CPAP**: These tests have made diagnosis and management of sleep apnea more affordable and effective. Sleep apnea is a root cause of heart attack, stroke, atrial fibrillation, hypertension and heart failure. Treating it can lower your risk of these events, lower your blood pressure, and reduce arterial inflammation.

- **Oral Microbiome Testing**: Oral microbiome testing involves taking a sample of saliva, and analyzing it to identify the types of bacteria present. If high risk bacteria that contribute to arterial inflammation are found, this can motivate more proactive management of periodontal disease, which contributes to heart attack and stroke risk.

  Knowing the nature of your oral "neighborhood" can prompt a more proactive approach to your oral hygiene. If there are dangerous criminals in your neighborhood, you will be more careful to "lock your doors" and augment your security for protection. Healthy gums decrease invasion, gingivitis, bacteremia and toxemia that can inflame arteries. The chronic diseases affected by your oral microbiome include periodontal disease, cardiovascular disease, Type 2 Diabetes and prediabetes, and even some cancers and dementia.

MY ULTRASOUND REVEALED ATHEROSCLEROSIS. WHAT'S NEXT?

If your screening ultrasound revealed atherosclerotic arterial disease, shown as "plaque," or inflammation in your artery wall, you can stop its progression and even reverse it, heal it and put it into remission. Improvement in the carotids, as measured by intima media thickness and reported as arterial age, predicts improvement in the coronary/heart arteries and elsewhere.

I'm often asked: "How can this be? How is it possible that I have arterial injury, inflammation and even plaque? How is it that doing everything I'm told is healthy still leaves me with this serious problem?"

Don't be offended. It isn't your fault. This happens quite often.

Sometimes the advice we are following is not optimal. A healthy lifestyle will prevent or slow the development of arterial injury from toxic food and lack of exercise, but it does not guarantee total protection. There are many factors that are lurking in the background that are overlooked by standard health care. You now have the opportunity to cover the blind spots, the gaps in your plan for a long healthy life. You can have safety and peace of mind.

This can include genetic factors that can be addressed to reduce the expression of these factors, vitamin D deficiency, homocysteine elevation due to inadequate folic acid, sleep disorders, stress, environmental toxins, insulin resistance (in spite of normal blood glucose levels) and others.

We identify these hidden root causes with our lab panel. Then we offer solutions to address revealed opportunities for greater safety and peace of mind, avoiding events, stents and surgery.

We measure the improvement and monitor to be sure that success is sustained with repeat lab testing, ultrasound to document improvement in arterial inflammation/age and body composition to follow reduction in body/visceral fat.

You can heal injury, inflammation and dangerous soft and heterogeneous plaque, driving plaque into stable and safe calcified plaque. Think of atherosclerosis like acne, an inflammatory condition of the skin with pimples that pop up in spots. Pimples and plaque are more prone to rupture right after they form. Pimple rupture creates a blood clot/scab to heal the rupture. A blood clot in the artery lumen blocks blood flow, causing damage to the tissue supplied by that artery. Coronary blockage results in heart attack or myocardial infarction. Carotid plaque rupture results in a stroke or transient ischemic attack. Both can be interrupted with rescue procedures, but proactive efforts to intervene and prevent events is far less risky and costly.

Stenosis or blockage, which affects blood flow capacity and chronic symptoms of angina or claudication, is much less important than the risk of plaque rupture, which is greatest with new soft plaque and least with old calcified plaque. Rupture suddenly appears as a stroke or heart attack.

These events are treated with emergency rescue care with stents and surgery. While waiting for treatment, you may suffer a fatal or life-altering stroke or cardiac arrest. You can also accumulate small silent strokes resulting in vascular dementia over time without noticeable acute symptoms.

These disasters can be avoided with proactive action to reverse disease into remission.

At the CureCenter, we strive to reverse atherosclerotic arterial inflammation, achieving remission to the point it is considered cured or healed, and no longer a threat. In other words, we Make Your Arteries Safe Again.

We collaborate and share results and recommendations with your current primary care provider and specialists who provide standard care. They may not understand all that we do. Even if they do, the system in which they practice blocks their ability to offer it. They may disagree, but they can't offer better.

We always welcome a conversation, especially if they will study our website or read "Healthy Heart Healthy Brain." Standard care tends to be reactive to symptoms and with procedural intervention, sometimes doing more harm than good. I always offer my mobile phone number to share with your doctor to discuss differences. It is rarely used.

Stents can fail, requiring further treatment and high-risk antiplatelet or blood thinners to prevent closure of the arteries. The CureCenter will help you get optimal results by creating a personalized lifestyle and medical CurePlan. We help you make changes you can live with. **We don't expect perfection. We support progress.**

MY ULTRASOUND DID NOT REVEAL ATHEROSCLEROSIS. WHAT NOW?

If your carotid ultrasound did not reveal significant atherosclerotic arterial injury/disease (seen as "plaque," or atheroma/inflammation in your artery wall), and your arterial age is significantly younger than your chronological age, that provides some peace of mind.

However, **there still may be disease in your coronary (or other) arteries**. The following recommendations become more relevant as you get older and with other common risk factors like family history of stroke, heart attack, stents or bypass surgery, high cholesterol, diabetes or prediabetes, high blood pressure, smoking or others. It is more important for a 60 year old with Type 2 Diabetes and hyperlipidemia than a 35 year old with few if any risk factors.

The next step in searching for arterial disease is finding your **Coronary Artery Calcium Score (CACS)**. *(If you've already had this test, we would be happy to review your results.)* Coronary Artery Calcium Score above zero means you have calcified atherosclerotic plaque/atheroma in your coronary arteries. Non calcified or homogeneous plaque/atheroma, which is the stage of plaque evolution that is the greatest risk for an event, is not detected by this test.

If you would like to find your CACS, do an internet search for "Coronary Artery Calcium Score near me" online. You should be able to find an imaging center or hospital that will offer this without a physician order. You can also call our office at 217-321-1987 or request a Discovery Zoom Call with Dr. Backs to discuss your results by visiting **theCureCenter.life**.

Beware: Coronary Artery Calcium Score is offered at a low entry price but is typically followed by recommendations for cardiology consultation, stress tests, echo-cardiograms and the slippery slope to stents and surgery. Before you accept invitations from the intervention focused cardiology program, schedule a Discovery Zoom Call to discuss your findings and options. The only stent any of my patients have needed was to fix the failure of a stent placed a couple of years earlier with no symptoms and for no evidence based benefit.

Of course, if you have had a stroke, TIA, heart attack, stent or surgery for vascular disease or other manifestation or proof of atherosclerosis/arterial disease, screening test results are not needed to get started.

WHAT IS A CORONARY ARTERY CALCIUM SCORE?

A coronary artery calcium scan reports your coronary artery calcium score. It is useful as a screening tool for those who are not known to have arterial disease. It should not be used to assess symptoms or monitor arterial disease in response to therapy.

If you already know of the presence of arterial disease in your body (if you've had a stroke, heart attack, stent, or bypass surgery) or carotid artery ultrasound, determining this score is unnecessary. It may also lead to risky, costly/profitable stents or surgery with no benefit in the absence of symptoms like angina or heart failure.

What does the score mean?

A score of zero is generally reassuring that the risk of heart attack from silent arterial disease is low in studied populations. You want this score to be as low as possible. However, if you have other risk or evidence of arterial disease, you could have plaque that is not calcified, known as soft/homogeneous/vulnerable/or unstable plaque. This occurs in about 10% of those with zero calcium scores.

Non-calcified plaque is the most vulnerable to rupture (the event that leads to heart attack). Therefore, a score of zero does not guarantee that you will not have a heart attack. Plaque can still form after a reassuring test in response to a change in conditions that promote inflammation, such as a dental infection or other inflammatory events.

Coronary calcium scores rise as plaque heals and inflammation subsides. In our experience, scores rarely fall, which makes this scan inappropriate for measuring improvement.

Instead, we recommend measuring trends of the thickness (sickness or inflammation) of your carotid arterial wall, which can be done with completely safe ultrasound. This is a much more meaningful measure of disease response to treatment. To find this option, visit vasolabs.com/events.

Coronary artery calcium scans can lead to a slippery slope that can be dangerous to your health and your pocketbook. They can lead to unnecessary procedures, such as stents, that do not prevent heart attack or stroke in individuals with no symptoms.

If there is no plaque seen on carotid ultrasound, an elevated Coronary Artery

Calcium Score should provoke a search for root causes and efforts to eliminate them.

The proper response to a positive screening/asymptomatic coronary artery calcium score should be to identify the root causes of arterial disease and eliminate them. This is the essence of a CurePlan from the CureCenter.

WHAT IS A CAROTID INTIMA MEDIA THICKNESS (CIMT) ULTRASOUND?

As part of your CurePlan, you will be urged to get a Carotid Intima Media Thickness (CIMT) ultrasound if possible. This is more detailed than the CureScreen carotid ultrasound process, carotid duplex ultrasound you can get at your hospital or vascular specialist or Life Line Screening. **It provides a much more detailed look at your artery wall and measures arterial inflammation**, which is the measurable and reversible underlying condition of interest.

Life Line screening identifies and encourages "monitoring" of plaque, but does not report intima media thickness for monitoring or offer a plan other than referral for surgery for late stage disease. It is useful for screening but not monitoring or proactive early intervention. If you have had a CureScreen ultrasound, you already have more information than a Life Line Screening ultrasound will offer, making it a waste of time and money better spent on a Carotid Intima Media Thickness ultrasound for disease monitoring.

Duplex ultrasound focuses on late stage flow restricting disease by focusing on blood flow velocity and lumen restriction. It ignores early disease, including the most dangerous homogeneous new plaque. Don't waste your time or money, even if covered by your insurance.

CIMT measures the thickness/inflammation of the artery wall and characteristics of plaque using ultrasound. It is typically repeated every 6-12 months. Trained medical, dental and other providers with Butterfly ultrasound probes can provide images sufficient for CIMT reports.

A thicker wall is a sicker, more inflamed wall with a higher risk of developing new unstable plaque. This inflammation, triggered by injury and oxidative stress from many sources, sets the stage for plaque development and rupture. Sudden unpredictable plaque rupture is the event leading to stroke and heart attack.

Having a little bit of arterial disease is like having a little bit of cancer. Like early cancer detection, our goal is to reverse arterial disease and achieve durable remission. When cancer remission is prolonged and stable, we think of it as cured. CIMT offers the most cost-effective, painless way to monitor progress toward a cure for arterial disease.

What is the difference between a CIMT and a duplex carotid ultrasound?

The CIMT offers more meaningful information about early arterial disease than standard duplex carotid ultrasound. It documents the type of plaque (estimating risk of rupture) and measures the thickness/inflammation of the artery wall.

The purpose of the duplex carotid ultrasound is to support the need for a surgical procedure by detecting late-stage disease while watching reversible early disease progress. Additionally, if you get a duplex ultrasound, your insurance likely won't pay for the more informative CIMT exam for at least six months. Many vascular labs mistakenly or misleadingly answer "yes" when asked if their ultrasound is a CIMT. The best bet is to go with one of the two providers nationwide that offer reliable and consistent CIMT testing at locations and times around the country: Vasolabs and Cardiorisk.

At the CureCenter, we depend upon the CIMT because it allows us to detect reversible early disease, assign an "arterial age," and show your improvement – something the duplex carotid ultrasound doesn't do. This added information and ability to track your progress will motivate your journey to optimize your CurePlan and rid yourself of chronic disease.

It is now possible to measure CIMT based on scans obtained by medical, dental and other professionals using point of care ultrasound supported by CureCoach, the Butterfly iQ ultrasound device and Vasolabs. Ask your dentist or doctor to consider this lifesaving opportunity for addition to their skill set and services.

What is arterial age?

The health of your carotid arteries reflects the health of arteries throughout your body, including the coronary arteries that supply blood to the heart. The carotid arteries are an accessible sample of a massive supply system.

Thickness of your artery wall is compared to other people your age and gender as a population percentile. Your "arterial age" is the age for which the thickness of your arteries would be average, i.e. 50th percentile. At the CureCenter, we monitor arterial age every 6-12 months to ensure our plan is working and your arterial age is improving. If it is not improving, we look for additional opportunities to improve your CurePlan.

Does Insurance Cover CIMT?

Medicare and most insurance covers CIMT if arterial disease is present, flow velocity measurements are included and performed by a certified sonographer.

This limits the number of providers who can offer this covered version. Cash payment options make it affordable for those with high deductibles or coverage only for catastrophic care.

It is now possible to provide equivalent relevant information using Butterfly point of care ultrasound in the hands of doctors, dentists, and others. This makes it more available at more times in more places. The scan is not payable by Medicare or insurance coverage because it doesn't meet their criteria. It is more than sufficient to detect disease and measure regression/improvement. The cost is $198, making it an affordable out of pocket expense compared to the cost of disability and death.

LIFE LINE SCREENING

Life Line Screening offers nationwide access to carotid artery ultrasound scanning for arterial disease. It is a good service that should be better. It calls attention to arterial disease and other signs of cardiometabolic disease. But it could have more impact than it does.

When they identify atherosclerotic disease, their recommendation to "monitor annually" supports the monitoring business plan but misses the best opportunity to reverse arterial disease when it is "mild."

Calling arterial disease "mild" is as logical as referring to "mild cancer." Would you accept a recommendation to monitor your early cancer and wait for advanced stage disease to intervene?

If the disease is advanced and they suggest referral to an interventional specialist, consider a Discovery Zoom Call with The CureCenter. But if you have even the earliest findings on your Life Line report in a drawer somewhere, we should have a discussion about it.

If you have a Life Line Screening report, register at **CureCoach.App**, then scan and upload the report to the message thread.

You can also fax your report to 866-594-7830 or mail a copy to The CureCenter for Chronic Disease, 2131 W. White Oaks Dr. Suite A, Springfield, IL 62704. Include contact information (mobile phone and email) so we can reach out to you.

We will review it and use it to advise you how it can motivate and support efforts to reverse your disease and get rid of the threat of stroke and heart attack by finding and mitigating your specific root causes with a personalized CurePlan.

YOU HAVE THE POWER: IMPROVE YOUR HEALTH

At the CureCenter, we believe that the best results come for those who engage to become empowered for better health. Diminish self-destructive choices and sustain better options. Do the best you can with what you have, forgive yourself when you fail, and get back on track longer after each failure.

Culture undermines and sabotages us. We are brainwashed by media and culture to eat addictive, poisonous junk and seek pleasure over purpose. We are encouraged to believe that our ills can be managed with pills and procedures that support the bottom line of the industries that profit from your chronic disease. You are not obliged to participate.

The person you can rely upon most is you. The CureCenter will give you the data, measurement and improvement tools and encouragement. We can coach you, but we can't play your game. You, the Player, will play out your CurePlan to win or lose.

Beware of saboteurs. They will be those closest to you who won't understand your plan and, intentions aside, encourage you to "have just one bite" because "I made this for you" and "everything in moderation." Your success may be their discomfort. It is easier to pull you back in than to escape their own choices.

Caretakers have a stake in the health of those for whom they care. We owe it to our loved ones to stay as healthy as possible, to not burden them with the consequences of a stroke or heart failure.

If there are barriers to success, we should acknowledge and seek ways to overcome them. Finances, time, responsibilities, and beliefs can stand in the way of success. Those we hang out with can drag us back from success if we challenge their choices. **Do not let the other crabs pull you back in the bucket.** Continue to inspire them to escape with you.

WHAT WILL MY PROVIDERS SAY ABOUT MY CUREPLAN?

Ideally, you should be able to trust your providers, from nurse practitioners to specialists, with your overall health and wellbeing. We all want to think of our doctor as "the best" and trust their advice.

Sadly, most "providers" are now employees of organizations that determine what they can and cannot offer. It is reasonable to ask, "Can I trust those who control my providers' paychecks who are influenced by financial imperatives?"

Here are some helpful questions to ask yourself when determining if your provider is right for you:

- What did my provider do to identify my chronic disease?
- What are they offering to CURE (not just manage) it?
- Do they wait and watch while it advances toward a more serious event such as heart attack or stroke?
- Do they offer you what they do for themselves?

When asked to detect "presymptomatic" arterial disease, most providers will schedule a stress test. The benefits of stress tests are only in the assessment of symptoms. They miss all but the most advanced state of coronary artery disease. False positives or equivocal tests lead to coronary angiograms and often unnecessary life altering stents.

Stop! Ask yourself, "How does this help me when I have no symptoms?" before agreeing to this approach. The only stent my patients have needed in the past 10 years was to fix the failure of a stent placed for a blockage in the absence of any symptoms. The other stent placed was done so in spite of measurement of no reduction in flow before stent placement.

For more information, we recommend reading the book *Prevention Myths* by Drs. Ford Brewer and Todd Eldredge.

Many modern providers are constrained by convention, guidelines, group think, complacency, and financial incentives to monitor and manage arterial and other chronic disease. They profit more from invasive, lucrative procedures and rehabilitation than they ever would from prevention. This is the business model that serves "health care" more than people. Surgery, stents and rehab are more profitable than healthy patients. **You are not the customer in this model. Your chronic disease is the product.**

This is not an attack on individual providers who work within the healthcare system, including your PCP and specialists. It is a sad observation of its brokenness and the corrupting nature of third party payment, employment of providers, and consolidation of healthcare into larger institutions. These institutions are dominated by those who have never uttered the Hippocratic Oath or watched a patient suffer in person.

You can do better.

At the CureCenter, we practice **Proactive Medicine. Most of us are past the point of prevention.** The tendency is to talk about prevention but act to fix a problem.

Our program reveals "presymptomatic" disease and "prevent" complications from progressive arterial disease. We expect to reverse your chronic disease and prevent untimely death or disability due to stroke, heart attack, or other major health events.

Side effects include feeling and looking better, more mental clarity and energy, and other positive effects. The goal is to live long, healthy, and happy and die old and healthy.

HOW DO I OPTIMIZE MY DIET FOR PREVENTION OF CHRONIC DISEASE?

The cause of most chronic diseases can be summed up using the Bad S's: Sweets, Starches, Snacks, Seed oils, Sitting, Smoking, Salt, Sleep Disturbance and Stress.

Should I go on a diet?

There are many diets: Paleo, Vegan, Ketogenic, Atkins, Zone, Mediterranean, Whole 30, Weight Watchers, and Nutrisystem to name a few. One of the main issues with dieting is that eventually you will go off, and then what happens? The whole plan falls apart and we typically regress to our original habits. The common promotion of eating three meals a day, "healthy" snacking, and counting calories create and perpetuate the problem. We are encouraged to graze like cows and eat to satisfy emotions. We are not well adapted to that behavior.

Our goal is to improve the way you view food and how it fits into your life and your health.

How can I optimize my diet without "dieting"?

- First, we recommend you **start with a baseline body composition analysis**. You improve what you measure. Don't be discouraged by your initial reading if it is not ideal. This measurement helps you set attainable goals and achieve them. The goals are incremental improvement, not some distant target.

  Weighing on a scale alone is not adequate. The body composition test allows you to know your muscle and fat mass, including your visceral fat. Visceral fat leads to diabetes and heart disease. Knowing this measurement is crucial to your overall health.

- **Come back regularly for additional body composition analyses.** Seeing "The Judge" for detailed, measurable improvement over time will help you stay motivated.

- **Drink more water.** Your urine should be copious and clear in appearance.

- **Avoid sweets (both natural and artificial).** There is added, hidden sugar in every processed food. Avoid them all!

  A rare sweet treat can be handled by most, but sugar is a toxin that should be avoided like tobacco. Processed food companies became the new employers for the scientists who increased the addictive nature of tobacco.

Artificial sweeteners raise insulin levels without raising glucose. Elevated insulin is the **most common** inflammatory stimulus, promoting prediabetes and arterial disease, among other chronic inflammatory conditions. These conditions dramatically flare when acute triggers, such as a virus or injury, cause additional inflammatory sickness. Artificial sweeteners are a "gateway drug" that strengthens your sweet tooth. They are a slippery slope to more sugar and carb cravings.

- **Avoid starches** including bread, pasta, white potatoes, and rice. Eat real food with no limits on vegetables, including sweet potatoes.
- **Limited amounts of fruit** provide micronutrients and fiber, but come with sugar. **Do not juice.** It removes fiber that makes the sugar in fruits absorb more slowly with less rise in insulin. **Avoid dried fruit,** as it is almost pure sugar.
- **Stop snacking.** Snacks are typically full of sugar and undermine our need to have periods of fasting to allow our insulin levels to drop. Fasting for 12-16 hours daily is a great "house cleaning" strategy.
- **Include good fats in your diet** such as olive oil, coconut oil, nuts, seeds, olives, and avocados. Include lean protein such as salmon, sardines, and poultry, in your diet. Eat red meat on a limited basis. When purchasing red meat, look for grass fed and organic options if you can afford them.
- **Intermittent fasting** (only drinking water, black coffee, and unsweetened tea) for 12-16 hours per day allows your insulin sensitivity to be regained by allowing your insulin levels to fall. I call it "window feeding" because you eat within a window or 6 hours as a goal.
- **Learn about the influence of your Microbiome.** While probiotic supplements may help, eating a prebiotic diet is even better. This includes fermented foods such as unpasteurized sauerkraut and Kim Chi. High fiber vegetables feed your good bacteria and can fix a great deal of health issues.
- **Get connected, motivated, and informed** to support your changes.

WHAT FOODS SHOULD I EAT AND WHAT SHOULD I AVOID?

At the CureCenter, we receive a lot of questions about diets, nutrition, and cooking. Therefore, we have put together some general advice and resources to help you improve your diet. We are happy to guide you through what you should be eating and what to avoid.

What types of foods should I eat?

- **Vegetables**: Try to eat as many different kinds of vegetables as possible (including sweet potatoes). A wide variety of plants provide essential and diverse nutrients. White potatoes and bread are starches, not vegetables.

- **Fruits**: While fruit is good for you and provides essential antioxidants, it also contains sugar. Therefore, it's important to limit the amount of fruit ingested on a daily basis. It is also good practice to try and eat a wide variety of fruits that offer different benefits. Instead of "fruits and vegetables" think "vegetables, vegetables, vegetables, some fruit, mostly berries." Bananas and grapes have too much sugar; avoid them.

- **Meat & Fish**: Protein is an important part of your diet and should not be overlooked. The protein you receive from meat should primarily come from fish, poultry and limited amounts of red meat. Fish, especially oily fish like salmon and sardines, are great sources of omega 3 fatty acids.

    When purchasing meat and fish, try to buy organic or wild caught, and not farm raised, if possible. Farm raised fish are fed grain, making them as unhealthy as corn fed beef. Eggs are also a great source of protein and good dietary cholesterol.

    If you are on a strictly plant based diet, make sure that you are supplementing for the protein and nutrients you won't be getting from meat, like B12. Starches are a problem for vegans. We see a lot of prediabetic potatoes and bread eating vegans.

- **Good Fats**: Consume good fats from olive oil, nuts, seeds, olives and avocados. Saturated fats, when consumed without high amounts of sugar in conjunction, do not increase the risk of heart disease or make you fat. Sugar is the culprit.

When should I eat?

We call it "window feeding." It is otherwise known as intermittent fasting or time restricted feeding.

Eat within as small a window of time every day as possible. Eight hours from your first food intake to your last is a good maximum window. Move the window around if possible: delay your first meal some days, then eat your last meal early other days.

Combined with a low sugar, low carb, whole food, plant-based goal, this lowers your overall insulin levels. Insulin elevation (hyperinsulinemia) is pro-inflammatory, which drives atherosclerosis and other chronic disease.

Why does this work? We are genetically best adapted to our remote ancestor hunter-gatherer pattern of alternating fasting and feasting. We don't thrive in our current "graze on sugary, processed food every waking hour of the day" culture.

Insulin resistance is a feature of our software for our hunter gatherer ancestors. Our grazing culture makes it a bug. In order to make it a feature, emulate the hunter gatherer eating pattern.

It also has emotional and spiritual benefits. To paraphrase Dr. Jason Fung, the only thing that Jesus, Abraham, Mohamed, Confucius, The Buddha, and every other religious movement leader agree upon is that fasting is good for us.

What types of foods should I avoid?

ASX10: Avoid Sweets, Starches, Snacks, Seed Oils.

Also Avoid Sitting, Salt, Smoking, Stress, Sleep deprivation
(On the contrary, Sex is a good thing for your health!).

- **Sweets/Added Sugar**: Refined sugar is the biggest contributor to inflammation and insulin resistance in our diets. Increases in the amount of sugar most Americans consume on a daily basis has gotten to absurd and dangerous levels. Sugar is causing the obesity, diabetes, and chronic disease epidemic that can easily be avoided with dietary changes. Added refined sugar is found most commonly in processed foods, including artificial sweeteners which can still cause an insulin response and sugar cravings.

- **Starch/Refined Carbohydrates**: Refined carbohydrates are found in highly processed breads, sweets, white potatoes, and processed snacks. The refined carbs break down into sugar and spike your insulin, making them dangerous to your overall health. Foods with high levels of refined carbs are stripped of many of their nutrients and contain a wide variety of chemicals used to increase their shelf life.

- **Sugary Drinks**: Do not drink beverages that have added sweeteners. Soda, sports drinks, energy drinks, sweetened tea, and coffee drinks all have large amounts of added sugar - both real and artificial. These drinks fuel insulin resistance, inflammation, obesity and tooth decay. Diet drinks are not better for you. They can raise insulin levels even without the calories. Low insulin levels are essential to avoiding chronic diseases such as diabetes.
- **Snacks/Processed Foods**: Avoid them. It is either "junk" or "food" but it can't be both. Stick to eating whole, unprocessed foods, not snack foods. Added sugar and preservatives make these products "addictive" and lead to long term health problems. Essential nutrients are taken out when these foods are being processed. Eat real food. Period.
- **Seed Oils**: Corn, sunflower, soybean and other vegetable oils are inflammatory. Use olive oil for cold applications. Use coconut, avocado and nut oils for hot cooking.

Do diets work?

There are numerous books and programs promoting diets. These diets may promise to transform your body in a given time frame, melt away fat, or promote other tactics that sound appealing and offer unusually rapid and effective results. The problem is that dieting is a temporary habit change which forces you to follow a system without teaching you how to improve your relationship to food.

Learn how good food fits into a healthier lifestyle that works for you.

Other Toxins:

While recent attention has been paid to micro-plastics, agricultural chemicals, dyes and other environmental toxins, it is difficult to detect them and modify your life enough on a daily basis long term. **Sugar is the most unnecessary and avoidable ubiquitous inflammatory environmental toxin.** Instead of worrying whether your Fruit Loops has a petroleum based red dye, avoid the dye and the sugar and other highly processed junk entirely by eating eggs and meat, not Fruit Loops, for breakfast. I suspect the sugar lobby is promoting the attention on these other toxins to divert attention from its role in chronic disease.

WHAT ARE HEALTHY WAYS TO COOK?

Truly healthy meals consist of whole unprocessed foods. The nutrients found in whole foods provide your body with all that it needs to maintain healthy body function and repair itself from illness and injury. How you prepare these foods also has an impact on your body's response. For example, deep frying vegetables in processed hydrogenated oil is not going to produce a healthy meal.

- **Start simple**: Cook basic meals made from healthy ingredients. Plan your meals around healthy options that are going to realistically fit into your lifestyle and allow you to consistently make good choices. There are many ways to modify recipes to remove bad ingredients and leave in nutrients, while maintaining the same good taste.
- **Change your mindset**: Healthy eating is not about going on a short term diet to drop a few pounds. The idea is to change your relationship with food and how you eat.
- **Plan ahead**: Set yourself up to succeed from the beginning to make healthy choices and not fall into a situation where you are choosing from only bad foods. Make sure you have meals planned out that include healthy options. Start bringing your lunch to work, cook dinner at home. Choose healthy options when you are eating out. Bring your own dressing for salads. Formulating a plan ahead of time will help you avoid bad decisions when you are hungry.

What are some healthy ways to modify recipes?

Choose olive oil for cold cooking and coconut oil for hot cooking. Avoid seed oils such as corn oil, soybean oil, sunflower oil, and others.

Use almond flour in place of wheat based flour. Cauliflower can be cooked and mashed or riced for a potato substitute. Sweet potatoes are healthier than white potatoes. Spaghetti squash is a good substitute for pasta.

What if I don't have time, resources, or willingness to cook?

Start simple with the resources you have. It may not lead to the most extravagant meals in the beginning, but the health benefits are worth it. Substitute frozen vegetables for canned foods. Empty your pantry and fill your refrigerator and freezer.

Consider meal delivery options, but be careful to do your research.

For those who are experienced in the kitchen, finding healthy recipes and modifying current ones will allow you to cook amazing meals that keep you healthy.

What are some good resources for finding healthy meal options?

This is not an exhaustive list, but includes resources that we have found helpful in discovering healthy recipes:

For Beginners:

- LearntoCook.com
- Food.com

For Diabetics:

- AllRecipes.com

Other Recipes:

- Healthy Eating | FoodNetwork.com/recipes
- Paleo Recipes | UltimatePaleoGuide.com

Other Helpful Resources:

- 25 Skills Every Cook Should Know | BBCGoodFood.com
- Vegan Diets: Practical Advice for Athletes & Exercisers | NIH
- EatReal.org
- NutritionCoalition.us

HOW CAN I USE CURECOACH.APP TO MEASURE MY NUTRITION?

CureCoach.App is our digital platform that supports our coaching effort to Cure Chronic Disease. When completing the Lifestyle Diet module, your answers provide you with tokens that are either green, yellow or red when viewing the summary page.

The answer options are "Rarely," "Sometimes," and "Frequently." Never should be reported as "rarely." For example, rare use of sugar and frequent consumption of vegetables gets you a green token. Frequent consumption of sugar and rare use of vegetables provoke red tokens. For those choices that are less clearly good or bad, you get a yellow token. Your goal over time is to increase the number of green tokens and decrease the number of red tokens by changing the choices and answers to these questions.

CureCoach.App can be accessed on your computer, tablet, or smartphone.

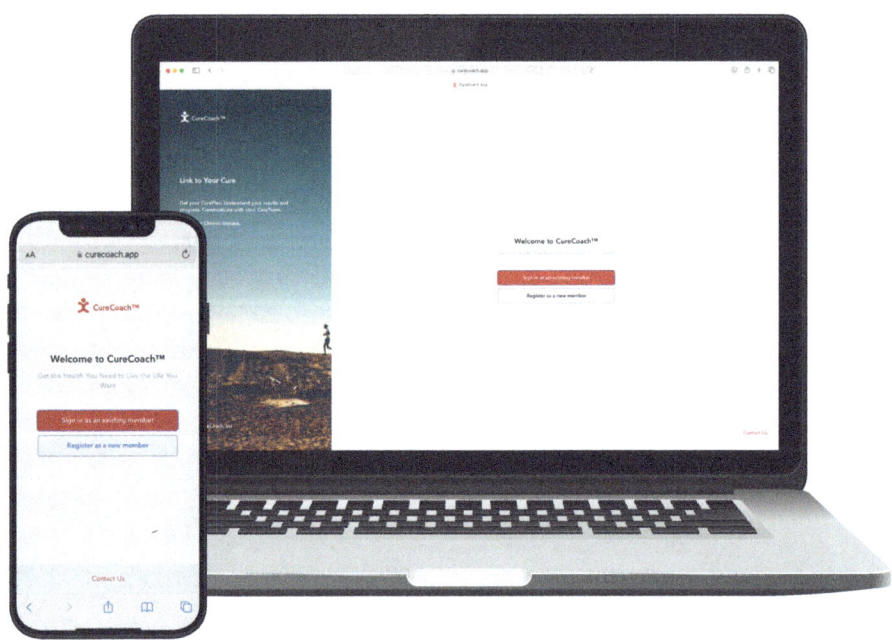

WHAT IS BODY COMPOSITION ANALYSIS?

Scales measure weight, which includes lean body mass, water, and fat. We urge you to go beyond the scale and get a body composition analysis, which measures your percent body fat and visceral fat.

We use the InBody 570. This machine reports visceral fat, which is the cause and effect of insulin resistance. Reduce visceral fat to reduce your insulin resistance, the most common root cause of arterial disease, diabetes, and prediabetes.

With the InBody 570, you can know exactly what you're made of: lean muscle mass, body fat mass, percentage of body fat, water, and visceral fat estimation, among other measurements. This will enable you to understand more completely the effects of the changes you make in your nutrition and exercise.

When you get a body composition analysis at the CureCenter, you will receive your results on **CureCoach.App**. Results over time are reported and pushed to your phone to monitor your progress. Our goal is to monitor visceral fat and percent body fat with the same interest as we monitor blood pressure and cholesterol. With our InBody technology, we can do this easily and frequently.

Measure, Mentor, Monitor, and Maintain Momentum. This is the key to your improvement.

Our body composition analysis is affordable. Insurers do not pay for this test. We don't want this to be a barrier.

Your initial InBody analysis is free of charge. Subsequent measurements are covered by our Proactive Medicine Membership.

WHAT IS VISCERAL FAT & HOW DO I REDUCE IT?

There are two types of fat that our body stores: subcutaneous fat and visceral fat.

Subcutaneous fat is stored just under the skin. We can pinch it in our arms, legs, and hips.

Visceral fat, or visceral adipose tissue, is the fat that is stored inside the body cavity and wraps itself around and infiltrates our internal organs, such as the heart, liver, or intestines. This fat is metabolically active and functions as if you had another organ in your body which produces negative hormonal effects. We call it "angry" or "inflammatory" fat.

Why is visceral fat dangerous?

Visceral fat is also referred to as "active" or "inflammatory" fat because it produces substances that contribute to insulin resistance, leading to Type 2 Diabetes. Insulin resistance is the prediabetic state where your body is losing its ability to properly balance insulin and regulate blood glucose.

Visceral fat secretes a protein called retinol-binding protein 4 (RBP4) that increases insulin resistance in the body. It also releases inflammatory substances called cytokines, which leads to chronic inflammation.

High levels of visceral fat are associated with increased risk for:

- Type 2 Diabetes
- Heart disease
- Breast cancer
- Colorectal cancer
- Alzheimer's disease
- Nonalcoholic fatty liver disease (NAFLD)

It is very difficult to be healthy with high amounts of visceral fat. Lowering visceral fat eliminates a major driver of chronic diseases.

What are the sources of visceral fat?

The root causes of visceral fat are refined carbohydrates, processed foods, and artificial sweeteners ingested without periods of fasting. This type of diet is typical in Western cultures. In order to eliminate visceral fat, the secret is to minimize the five S's: Sweets, Starch, Snacks, Seed oils, and Sitting.

How do you test for visceral fat?

There are many ways to estimate your visceral fat. MRI, DEXA, and CT scans are accurate but costly and inconvenient. A cheaper way to estimate visceral fat is to measure your waistline. A healthy waistline in women is typically 35" or lower, and 40" or lower for men. However, these measurements are prone to variability. They are inexpensive, but not precise.

At the CureCenter, we have a simple, non-invasive, and cost-effective way to measure and monitor visceral fat. We use the InBody 570 analyzer to obtain accurate body composition data on our patients repeatedly over time. This data allows us to monitor not only visceral fat, but percent body fat, skeletal muscle mass, and hydration levels. This information is crucial in monitoring the benefit of our treatment and demonstrating optimal results. The InBody data goes far beyond the scale and helps us provide motivation for ongoing lifestyle improvements.

Body composition tests using the InBody 570 only take a few minutes and are completely painless and non-invasive. The process is similar to stepping on a scale - only this machine measures much more than your average at-home device. If you have a pacemaker or defibrillator, or you are pregnant, we don't use the InBody, even though the risk is not high.

How do I eliminate visceral fat?

- **Reduce your sugar intake**, especially sugary drinks, refined white carbohydrates, and processed foods.
- **Avoid artificial sweeteners.** They raise insulin in the same way as sugar, even though they are lower in calories. They also perpetuate cravings for real sugar by feeding your sweet tooth, like a "gateway" drug.
- **Restrict eating to a window of time** (ideally 6-8 hours) and devote time every day to fasting (drinking only water or non-sugary drinks). At least 16 hours of fasting, including sleep, is a goal we promote to our patients. We call it "window feeding."
- **Exercise** as much as you can most days.
- **Eat a low-glycemic diet.** Low-glycemic foods consist of green vegetables, whole fruits (in moderation), beans, and lentils.
- **Get a good night's sleep.** Too little sleep or too much sleep on a regular basis can lead to more visceral fat storage.

- **Manage stress.** Mindfulness practices like prayer, meditation, or yoga can help manage your body's stress response and lower cortisol levels.
- **Limit alcohol.** When your liver is processing alcohol, it is not processing fat.
- **Quit smoking.** Tobacco use can negatively affect your ability to deal with glucose and increase insulin resistance.
- **Targeted supplements and medications** can improve insulin sensitivity for some individuals with stubborn visceral fat.

WHAT IS CONTINUOUS GLUCOSE MONITORING (CGM)?

At The CureCenter, we understand that dealing with insulin resistance, prediabetes and diabetes can be an ongoing struggle that comes with a wide range of issues, including:

- Trying to reach A1C goals
- Experiencing low blood sugar
- Not being able to control highs after eating
- Wondering how food is affecting your blood glucose
- Find the right medication and dosage if lifestyle optimization needs help

This is why we support Continuous Glucose Monitoring (CGM) for our patients with Type 2 Diabetes, prediabetes and those who exhibit chronic inflammation from insulin resistance.

A CGM is a device that continuously measures the levels of glucose in the blood. It works through a small sensor that is inserted through the skin and is connected to a transmitter which sends glucose readings to a receiver or app. It can provide real-time reporting about an individual's blood-glucose levels.

Insights from these reports make a real difference in the management of our patients with insulin resistance. They help us learn the impact of everyday decisions about diet and exercise and gain insights into the effects of medication changes.

CGM is a very powerful tool to optimally manage and control insulin resistance, one of the most common root causes for arterial disease.

What type of CGM do you use at the CureCenter?

At the CureCenter, we prescribe the devices most available to you. It is a cost-effective alternative to ketone metering and finger sticks for blood glucose monitoring for those who want to reduce their risk of diabetes and other chronic diseases.

For less than $5 per day for 28 days, you can continuously measure your blood glucose response to your food and other behavior choices with a CGM.

You will need a prescription for this CGM. If you are not taking insulin, your insurance will not cover it. However, it is affordable and the benefits of the data are priceless.

WHAT IS THE DIFFERENCE BETWEEN A CUREPLAN AND THE ORNISH REVERSAL PROGRAM?

Years ago, after taking advantage of our CureScreen carotid ultrasound to detect plaque, a patient declined our help. He thought our program was the same as the Ornish Reversal Program, in which he had already been participating. This, however, is not true.

Over the years, we've had at least three patients who have compared our program to Ornish. Two of them chose the CureCenter and have shown measurable improvement. The third completed the Ornish Reversal Program with deterioration in his diabetes control. Turns out a whole food plant based diet can have a lot of starch that turns into sugar. He made an appointment to come back to the CureCenter. Sadly, he died in his sleep before his appointment.

Our plan is not the same as the Ornish Reversal Program. We think it is a better alternative for most.

What is the Ornish Reversal Program?

The Ornish Reversal Program improves health through lifestyle modifications that prevent or reverse heart disease. Although, on the surface, it sounds similar to the CureCenter's program, it doesn't address the role of sweets, starches, and snacks that can be very dangerous to your health.

What are some differences between this program and the CureCenter's program?

Below is a list of some major differences in philosophy between the Ornish Reversal Program and the CureCenter's Cureplan:

- **CurePlan**: Focuses on inflammation as a root cause of atherosclerosis.
- **Ornish Program**: Barely addresses inflammation.

- **CurePlan**: Encourages plant-focused nutrition and consumption of good fats. Limits sweets, starches, and snacking. Promotes Time Restricted Feeding (also known as intermittent fasting). We call it "window feeding."
- **Ornish Program**: Encourages a diet unrestricted in carbohydrates and low in protein and good fats.

- **CurePlan**: Promotes oral health as a priority for arterial health.
- **Ornish Program**: No mention of the role of oral inflammatory disease - a driver of arterial inflammation and a contributor to as many as 50% of strokes and heart attacks.

- **CurePlan**: Uses genetic testing to personalize your CurePlan.
- **Ornish Program**: No personalization based on genetic testing.

- **CurePlan**: Offers manageable nudges in the direction of simple solutions you can live with and accountability through measurement and feedback. Simple solutions are more sustainable and effective than radical complex solutions. Measurement supports success.
- **Ornish Program**: Requires strict adherence to a vegetarian diet and 72 hours of class attendance that may be difficult to schedule and complete.

The Ornish Program has financial relationships with McDonald's and other manufacturers of highly processed, carbohydrate-rich foods. They sell the root cause of Type 2 Diabetes and heart disease, even in their so-called "healthy" options.

The CureCenter interests align with your interest. We both benefit from your longevity and improved quality of life for a long healthy relationship.

The Ornish program is full of **activity**. Your CurePlan is focused on **accomplishment**.

You will decide which is a better fit for you and your life.

HOW DOES VITAMIN D DEFICIENCY AFFECT MY HEALTH?

Vitamin D is an important nutrient, actually a hormone, that helps the body absorb and bind calcium, which is essential for maintaining strong bones and teeth. It also plays a role in the immune system, muscle function, and reduction of inflammation. Optimal levels of vitamin D are above 50ng/ml. Don't let anyone convince you that this can be "too high" and to stop your supplement. They don't know the benefits of vitamin D levels above the population normal because the population as a whole is deficient.

Up to 75% of Americans are affected by suboptimal vitamin D, which significantly increases the risk of heart attack, stroke, hypertension, diabetes, cognitive impairment, and cancer. Having darker skin, being obese, and not getting enough sun exposure to the skin are all linked to reduced vitamin D3 levels.

Symptoms of vitamin D deficiency include muscle pain, tiredness, fatigue, hair loss, back pain, bone loss, poor wound healing, and depression. It increases the risk of statin muscle pain. However, most individuals who are vitamin D deficient have no specific symptoms.

What causes vitamin D deficiency?

- **Inadequate sun exposure.** Sunlight is the optimal source of vitamin D. When the skin is exposed to UVB radiation from sunlight, it produces a form of vitamin D known as cholecalciferol, or vitamin D3. Vitamin D3 is then converted into its active form in the liver and kidneys. This particularly affects individuals who are in institutions like nursing homes.
- **Dark skin.** Melanin, the pigment that gives skin its color, reduces the skin's ability to produce vitamin D in response to sunlight. Melanin absorbs UVB radiation from sunlight, which is needed for the skin to produce vitamin D. This means that people with darker skin require more sun exposure to produce the same amount of vitamin D as people with lighter skin.
- **Old age.** The skin's ability to produce vitamin D declines with age due to a variety of factors, including a reduced ability to convert sunlight to vitamin D, decreased skin thickness, and lower levels of the precursor molecules that are needed to produce vitamin D.

- **Obesity.** Vitamin D is a fat-soluble vitamin, meaning it is stored in fatty tissues. Therefore, people with higher levels of body fat may require more vitamin D to achieve the same blood levels as people with lower levels of body fat.
- **Diseased kidneys.** The kidneys are important for converting vitamin D into a form that the body can use. If the kidneys are not working well due to a disease, they may not be able to convert vitamin D properly, leading to a deficiency of vitamin D in the body.
- **Digestive tract issues** (such as Crohn's disease, celiac disease, or cystic fibrosis). Vitamin D is a fat-soluble vitamin, which means it needs to be absorbed in the presence of dietary fat in the small intestine. Digestive tract issues can affect the absorption of vitamin D in the small intestine. These conditions can cause inflammation or damage to the intestinal lining, which can interfere with the absorption of dietary fat and, consequently, vitamin D.
- **A vegan diet without proper supplementation.** Vitamin D is primarily found in animal-based foods such as fatty fish, liver, and egg yolks. Therefore, people following a strict vegan diet that avoids all animal products are at risk of vitamin D deficiency.
- **Sunblock.** When the skin is exposed to ultraviolet (UV) radiation, it triggers the synthesis of vitamin D3, which is then used by the body. However, using sunblock or sunscreen can reduce the skin's ability to produce vitamin D, as it blocks the UV radiation from penetrating the skin. It's important to find a balance between protecting your skin from harmful UV radiation and ensuring adequate vitamin D levels.

How can I treat vitamin D deficiency?

- **Increase sun exposure.** Make an effort to get a healthy amount of sun exposure without putting yourself at risk for skin damage or skin cancer. It's recommended to get a moderate amount of sun exposure, typically around 10-15 minutes per day, without sunscreen, on the arms, legs, and face.
- **Eat vitamin D rich foods.** Foods that are rich in vitamin D include salmon, sardines, tuna, egg yolks, fortified milk, and shiitake mushrooms.
- **Vitamin D supplements.** Supplementation can bring your levels into the optimal range. We recommend a combination of Vitamin D3 and Vitamin K2. Vitamin K2 enhances vitamin D absorption, delivery, and the binding of Vitamin D3 in the appropriate tissues, enhancing its activity and benefit. Vitamin K2 also improves arterial elasticity and insulin sensitivity. The product we stock and recommend is called "K Force."

How do I know if I've properly treated my vitamin D deficiency?

Get a blood test measuring the serum concentration of 25(OH)D3. A "normal" level of vitamin D is at least 30ng/mL or higher. However, our "optimal" range is 60-90ng/ML.

If you have been diagnosed with vitamin D deficiency and have started taking supplements or made changes to your diet, get your vitamin D levels retested after a few months.

ARE SUPPLEMENTS BENEFICIAL?

As a traditional allopathic physician, Dr. Backs was trained to be skeptical of supplements. That has changed. He is now a more "open minded" allopath. There is evidence to support the use of supplements for specific purposes.

How do I know what supplements I should take?

The supplement industry is largely unregulated, which means you should be careful about the source of supplements you take. Here are some tips to avoid supplements that can damage your health and budget:

- Choose products from companies that validate the content of their products by submitting to FDA monitoring for content.
- Look for evidence from clinical trials when they are available.
- Don't rely solely on the recommendation of a friend who sells you a product and then engages you as a promoter of the product. These multi level marketing schemes generally benefit the founders at the expense of later entrants.
- Don't hide the use of supplements from your physicians. They can interact with other drugs and influence your treatment. If you have stopped taking them, share that and the reason for stopping them. If the issue is cost, we can look at alternatives. But we can't do our best if information is incomplete, whatever the motivation.
- We use Fullscript to provide easy online access to plans and recommend specific supplements that are high value at a fair price.

Here is a list of some of the common supplements we recommend at the CureCenter and their benefits:

- **Bergamot BPF**: Extracted from the Bergamot lime/orange through a special process, this food extract has been shown to have many of the beneficial effects of statins (reduce LDL and inflammation) while also improving insulin sensitivity, the underlying cause of Type 2 Diabetes. We have also found it to be correlated with reduced lipoprotein(a) in some cases. We recommend it commonly for those who don't tolerate statins, who need its help for insulin resistance or prefer non pharmacologic treatments for arterial disease and hyperlipidemia. We often recommend it to synergize with statins for even more improvement in lipids and insulin resistance.

- **Niacin (Vitamin B3)**: At the CureCenter, we recommend timed or slow release niacin for those with elevated Lipoprotein(a) and small dense LDL dyslipidemia. For those who can't or won't take statins, it has favorable effects on lipids and inflammation. There are benefits to taking Niacin that make it worthwhile despite dealing with some annoying effects, including flushing. Taking it at bedtime makes it more tolerable by sleeping through the flush. Diphenhydramine can help minimize the flushing experience. Others use its warming effect prior to workouts. To each its own.

- **Vitamin D3**: This supplement addresses our all-too-common deficiency of vitamin D. "Normal" levels of vitamin D3 (>30) are not optimal. Our target is a level of 60-90. Toxicity is not a problem until well above a level of 100.

    At the CureCenter, we recommend vitamin D3 with vitamin K2. K2 serves as a transport/binding agent for vitamin D that enhances its effectiveness. Vitamin K2 also has potential arterial elasticity promoting properties, and improves insulin sensitivity. Click here for more information about vitamin K2. While there is talk about K2 "removing" calcium from arteries, it is more accurate to claim that less plaque is created when we improve insulin sensitivity and chronic inflammation with K2

- **Diaxinol**: This supplement combines a number of agents that enhance insulin sensitivity (reduce insulin resistance). Cinnamon can be a lower-cost alternative, but with the concentrated cinnamon extract and other agents in Diaxinol, we see more consistent improvement in measures that reflect insulin resistance.

- **Fish Oil (Omega 3 fatty acids)**: These supplements act to lower inflammation, reduce platelet adhesion, and have several favorable effects on lipids. Our goal is to get about 200mg of combined DHA (docosahexaenoic acid) and EPA (eicosapentaenoic acid) daily. They also have an anticoagulant effect so be aware of increased bleeding risk, especially if taking aspirin or other antiplatelet or anticoagulant drugs.

- **Turmeric (curcumin)**: This is a spice with anti-inflammatory benefits that can also be taken in supplement form. Since atherosclerosis is an inflammatory disease, the potential benefits are worth considering.

- **Vitamin E**: This vitamin improves arterial event (heart attack, stroke, etc.) risk in patients with Haptoglobin genotype 2-2 while increasing the risk for those whose genotype is 1-1 or 1-2. We recommend natural alpha-tocopherol vitamin E (400 IU daily) but only after documenting your haptoglobin genotype.

- **Ubiquinol or CoEnzyme Q 10**: This supplement may mitigate statin muscle pain side effects and are recommended for anyone on a statin, especially those on higher doses.

    Probiotics and a Prebiotic diet improves the gut microbiome, which interacts with the human body in ways that are only in the beginning stages of study and understanding. The gut microbiome can be harmed by antibiotics and environmental agents that act to alter the microbiome. Probiotics can help maintain and restore the good bacteria that we depend upon for good health. A better alternative is a "prebiotic" diet with lots of vegetable fiber and fermented foods like unpasteurized sauerkraut and kim chi.

At the CureCenter, our recommendation of specific products is intended to assure that our patients get reliable benefits at a fair price. We want you to get what you pay for. We connect you with Fullscript to enable convenient home delivery while supporting our efforts to get the correct supplement and a good value.

STATINS: THE REST OF THE STORY

There is a rise in the religion of "antistatinism." Another way to put it: There is a "War on Statins." Just like there was a war on early treatment of a serious viral illness with safe repurposed medication. I prefer to share a positive fact based message.

But I must fight back to promote optimal outcomes and maximize quality and quantity of life. If antistatinism is your religion, no need to read further. You won't be convinced by data or admit you might have been fooled. I can't coach someone who already knows everything.

But many are struggling with the threat of disability or death vs the propaganda designed to lure you to drive your money to their "solution" and their profit.

I'm frustrated almost daily by patients when, in addition to prescribing healthier lifestyle and correction of deficiencies, I explain the benefits and reversible risks and prescribe statins while monitoring for their benefit and harm. They are stable or improving on very well tolerated low dose rosuvastatin but stop this life saving treatment in spite of demonstrated life threatening atherosclerosis with measurable personal improvement in inflammation, arterial age, plaque healing and inflammatory markers because of "something I've read."

I don't blame the patients. We are susceptible to "fear porn" propaganda. I blame the opportunistic writers who are pushing people toward far more costly and more profitable PCSK9 inhibitors, expensive and less effective nutraceuticals, stents, surgery, cardiac/stroke rehab, dialysis, memory care centers and funeral expenses in their pursuit of likes, followers, and speaking fees based more on charisma and charm than interest in you personally!

Every one of these messengers has a business plan counting on growth!

Everything must be read with a filter of "what is offered as an alternative and what is the financial conflict of interest?" And "what does the author know or care about my individual circumstances, results and needs?"

I get it, but let's put facts before feelings on this issue. Are statins mis/over prescribed? For sure. Is it driven by profit motive? It's hard to blame this when almost all statins are cheap generics. Mostly, the driver is the guidelines that employed providers must follow and check the box under financial incentives and penalties to adhere. Reducing arterial disease progression or achieving remission doesn't support a multi-billion dollar procedural intervention and rehabilitation business model projecting and depending on growth. This is why I'm suspicious of any interventional cardiologist who disputes efforts to achieve remission, including statins to reduce inflammation. I'd prefer to hear more about the useless and potentially harmful stents placed over the years in asymptomatic individuals provoked by the "oculostenotic reflex" and provider revenue incentives.

Statin fear drives demand for more profitable pharma options like PCSK9 inhibitors (more than $500/month vs $5/month for generic rosuvastatin on GoodRx) and nutraceutical alternatives.

Statins are the most proven pharmaceutical treatment (in addition to a healthy diet and exercise) for remission of arterial disease and the reduction of heart attack and stroke for those with arterial injury/disease/plaque.

Evidence strongly supports that statins prevent death and disability from heart attack and stroke in patients with arterial disease. That evidence guides us to recommend statins at lower but still effective and well tolerated doses for those with atherosclerosis, which we identify and measure using carotid ultrasound and coronary calcium scoring. We monitor inflammation levels with ultrasound (intima media thickness measurement) and blood tests: C reactive protein, LpPLA2, microalbumin/creatinine ratio and myeloperoxidase. We consistently see improvement in these measures on statins and deterioration when stopped. I recently documented an 18 year improvement in arterial age in less than 5 months in a 66 year old clean living man while on rosuvastatin 5 mg 3 times weekly in addition to his continued healthy lifestyle. It is common for patients to admit to stopping their statin when confronted with mysterious adverse results on these measures after maintaining they were adherent prior to seeing the numbers. The numbers don't lie!

You should be far more afraid of untreated inflamed plaque killing or disabling you than concerns about reversible annoying symptoms from an inexpensive generic medication that offers reliable protection. There is little controversy about statin benefit after an event (heart attack, stroke, bypass surgery or stent). When we find plaque (ultrasound or coronary calcium score) we consider those findings as essentially a near miss, an event that, fortunately, did not cause damage. Next time plaque develops, you might not be so lucky.

The foundation of health is nutrition/lifestyle/toxin avoidance. Think of this as the "belt" that keeps our pants from falling down. Statins are like "suspenders" that cover our lapses in optimal lifestyle choices. Safety programs, like airlines and the space program, are built on redundancy and backup plans. Belts AND Suspenders provided by the Department of Redundancy Department.

What is the primary source of negative information about statins?

The biggest problem with statins is higher than needed doses of the wrong statin prescribed for the wrong reason. This is particularly true of the least effective but most effectively marketed statins (e.g. atorvastatin) for the lowering of LDL to target cholesterol levels based on general guidelines. The focus should be on reduced inflammation as measured by LpPLA2, myeloperoxidase and intima media thickness/arterial age by ultrasound in the individual.

At the CureCenter, **we don't prescribe statins if the arteries are healthy**, no matter how "bad" the cholesterol is. We prescribe lower doses of rosuvastatin (has shown the strongest evidence of reduction in cardiovascular events while not crossing the blood brain barrier or promoting diabetes) based on documented atherosclerotic arterial plaque or inflammation, identification and monitoring of LpPLA2, myeloperoxidase and carotid intima media thickness/arterial age.

Event risk reduction begins in hours, but not for the reason most think. Statins lower LDL cholesterol levels, but their most potent benefit is reduced inflammation in the artery wall. I have seen this repeatedly by monitoring LpPLA2 and carotid intima media thickness trends.

Statin adherence consistently yields improvement. I can tell when they have been stopped by unfavorable trends in LpPLA2 and CIMT. In other words, they stabilize/heal plaque and improve the health and age of diseased arteries! There is evidence they reduced COVID deaths, probably due to suppression of baseline inflammation and mitigating the inflammatory effect of spike protein. Is it possible they protect my from vaccine injury as well?

When encountering negative propaganda about statins, ask the following questions:

- Is the alternative offered a more expensive and profitable proprietary supplement or pharmaceutical? Statins should cost less than $10/month and are usually covered by insurance. Supplements will cost 2-4 times that amount and not covered by insurance. Ezetimibe is less effective at reducing inflammation. PCSK9 cost more than $500/month. To get coverage, it helps if you are "statin intolerant" which can be promoted by the "nocebo" effect. They cannot claim superior results except with extreme familial hyperlipidemia. But that would make them "orphan drugs. Pharma prefers blockbuster profits.

- Does the reduction or elimination of heart attack, stroke, bypass surgery, stents, and rehab for heart attack and stroke undermine their business plan and revenue from treating late stage disease with stents, surgery, rehab, dialysis, memory care centers and funeral expenses?
- Is the goal reduction of cholesterol or prevention of heart attack, stroke, premature death, surgery, stents or rehab by suppressing inflammation due to oxidative stress?
- Is the advisor using the optimal measurement tools that show improvement in arterial health/age as we do at The CureCenter with Carotid Intima Media Thickness ultrasound or blood markers of arterial inflammation? Or are they solely focused on LDL cholesterol?
- Is the advisor like a child with a hammer pounding on everything that looks like a nail? Are they using all the tools and options available from a program in pursuit of optimal quality of life and longevity?

How does the CureCenter prescribe and measure the benefits of statin use?

When prescribing statins, the only reason we monitor lipid levels is that we are expected to do so AND as a way to verify that the medication is being taken. We measure benefit by demonstrating a reduction in measures of inflammation and arterial wall thickness using CIMT.

In some cases, we will pay less attention to elevated cholesterol levels if we know that arteries are healthy based on healthy carotid ultrasound and coronary calcium score.

In other cases, if we know that arteries are sick in spite of normal cholesterol levels, we generally prescribe statins unless we know of prior intolerance based on personal experience. Arteries improve with statins in spite of "normal" cholesterol because statins reduce inflammation. We generally use lower doses of statins (fewer side effects) because we are treating for artery health improvement, not the lowest possible LDL cholesterol levels.

Has Dr. Backs had his own personal experience with statin use?

Dr. Backs personally takes a daily statin called rosuvastatin. When he stopped it for a time (to see if his muscles ached from hard workouts or the drug), his arterial age increased by 10 years while he experienced the same sore muscles. This is all while he continued to exercise and live the "cleanest" lifestyle possible.

When the statin was resumed, the arterial age returned to lower levels.

Do statins have any side effects?

Statins can provoke dose dependent side effects in a minority of users most commonly muscle aching. The vast majority of individuals can take them safely with benefit with no adverse results. Untreated sleep apnea and low vitamin D levels increase the likelihood of muscle aches. Correction of these issues reduces these side effects and has other benefits. Coenzyme Q may be helpful, but reducing the dose of the statin or changing to a better tolerated option is the best first step for someone whose arteries are a threat.

A small minority of users have reported cognitive harm in relation to statins. This is less likely with rosuvastatin, our preference, because it does not cross the blood brain barrier like Lipitor/atorvastatin, the most successfully marketed statin.

Reduction in arterial disease-related dementia is far greater than the incidence of reversible cognitive compromise from statins. If you experience cognitive changes after starting a statin, they will reverse when the drug is stopped if due to the statin. Don't get stuck on this worry. Dementia and Alzheimer's are a far greater risk with arterial disease and insulin resistance driven chronic inflammation. Therefore, addressing this risk is far more important than fearing a temporary side effect.

Increased diabetes risk and insulin resistance have also been a concern. In many cases, patients are not counseled to or fail to reduce sweets and starches in their diets, thinking they are protected by the statin prescription. In fact, the focus on salt, fat and cholesterol leads to increased inflammatory addicting sugar intake. Therefore, it is no wonder that they progress from insulin resistance to prediabetes to Type 2 Diabetes, the progression caused by the western processed glycemic diet. Reduced Sweets, Starches and Snacks in the diet can offset fears about increased risk of diabetes or insulin resistance. Our patients are constantly coached and monitored for evidence of progression to prediabetes or Type 2 Diabetes.

Without personally trying a drug, predicting how you will tolerate it is impossible! The experience of a friend or family member, while provoking understandable concern and fear, will not predict your experience with statins or any other drug. Fears of statin intolerance tend to be self-fulfilling. This is known as the "nocebo" effect.

Intolerance of one statin doesn't necessarily predict intolerance of all statins. Some side effects disappear with lower doses that will still have benefit measurable by blood and ultrasound measurements of inflammation.

At the CureCenter, we monitor reaction to any medication we recommend, both good and bad. Our bottom line: If you have atherosclerosis, you will generally benefit from a statin (if you can tolerate it) to reverse arterial inflammation, heal plaque and prevent life altering events: heart attack, stroke, and dementia.

If you are still skeptical, we offer alternatives like Bergamot BPF or niacin. None of these have the same degree of net favorable track record of statins, and side effects are not zero. They offer benefits that vary by individual.

Open minded willingness to consider risks AND benefits of any treatment leads to the best outcomes. But if your mind is made up, and you decline to take a statin, we won't "have a stroke" over it.

We hope and pray the same is true for our patients.

WHY IS ORAL HEALTH IMPORTANT TO MY OVERALL HEALTH?

Oral health has a bigger impact on your overall health than you likely suspect. Inflammation and disease in the mouth can have a negative impact throughout your whole body and lead to some very serious conditions. **Bacterial, viral and fungal pathogens contribute to arterial disease** (50% of heart attacks and strokes!) metabolic disease (insulin resistance, prediabetes, Type 2 Diabetes), cancer, dementia, high risk pregnancy, and inflammatory arthritis.

One of the key players in this oral systemic connection are the bacteria in your mouth. There are both good and bad bacteria that inhabit the mouth, the "oral microbiome." The goal is to maintain barriers to invasion locally (gingivitis and periodontitis) and systemically (arterial injury) reduce the population of the bad bacteria and create an environment to promote good bacteria.

While colonization is difficult or impossible to eliminate, **prevention of infection of gums and systemic invasion are the primary goals of an optimal oral hygiene routine**. Brushing and flossing are the foundation of good oral hygiene, but may not be enough if bad bacteria have taken hold. Your dentist and hygienist are the best source for your plan.

How are bad bacteria detected?

Visual inspection alone will not pick up the presence of high risk bacteria. Even if your gum tissues appear healthy, these bacteria may invade subtle pockets of inflammation or be opportunistic for a lapse in hygiene or the barrier to invasion associated with healthy gums. This can turn colonization into infection and inflammation in the gums, arteries and elsewhere.

More and more dentists and hygienists are highlighting the connection between the mouth and the rest of the body. If your dental care providers are on board with this focus, you are fortunate. If your dentist is unaware or uninterested in this connection, The CureCenter can recommend oral health providers who are on board for at least a second opinion and perhaps a transfer of care.

We use saliva testing to measure the amount of bad or pathogenic bacteria in the mouth. The results will motivate a plan (provided by a dental professional) to address the concern. The key is to reduce the level of bad bacteria that contribute to chronic disease and preserve barriers to invasiveness locally and systemically. For more detail, click SimplyPerio. In general, we classify Fn as "bad, Td and Tf as "worse" and Pg and Aa as "the worst" bacteria to be present in the mouth.

What should my dentist be looking for?

Dentists who are on the leading edge of oral care use cone beam/3D CT scans to look for presymptomatic abscesses and other issues that may be missed by routine examination and standard x-rays. These conditions don't always cause symptoms that would cause concern. This can be dangerous because the first noticeable symptom could be a heart attack or stroke. High risk oral pathogens can also contribute to poor control of diabetes and prediabetes.

We recommend cone beam CT, especially for our patients who have had prior events or elevated myeloperoxidase (MPO). Traditional x-rays will routinely miss abscesses that could be driving arterial inflammation and increase the likelihood of heart attack or stroke. For example, old root canals can be sites of chronic inflammation but detection may not be possible without use of the cone beam CT.

At the CureCenter, we will work with your current dentist to gather this type of information if they show an interest. If not, we can recommend a dentist who we know is on board with this process.

What can I do to avoid oral health issues?

Choose a dental professional who understands concerns beyond your teeth. You can find this out by learning if your dentist has participated in continuing education about the oral systemic connection. Regularly visit this dental professional and make sure they provide an ongoing treatment plan for any issues. Follow their plan.

Get saliva testing at least once to discover any bad bacteria that may be present. We have seen patients that have no obvious issues or new cavities that have had significant levels of dangerous bacteria in spite of their current dental plan. Don't let colonization with these bacteria become invasive infection in your gums or arteries.

Associations between high risk (red complex) oral bacteria and serious medical conditions and complications.

Follow a daily routine to maintain proper oral care and prevent bad bacteria from growing in your mouth. Daily brushing and flossing can be augmented with use of a waterpik and dental picks. Use a pH neutral mouth rinse twice daily to help promote healthy bacteria that protect teeth and gums. Brush your entire mouth, not just the teeth and gums, and always go to bed with a clean mouth.

During the day, choose 100% xylitol gum or mints and eat tooth protecting foods (low carb/high protein) at the end of meals or snacks.

HR5 Pathogen/Condition Associations

Condition/Pathogen	Aa	Pg	Td	Tf	Fn
Heart Disease	●	●	●	●	○
Ischemic Stroke	●	●	●	●	
Alzheimer's/Dementia	●	●	●	●	○
Brain Abscess	●				
Aneurysm	●	●	●	●	
Atherosclerosis	●	●	●	●	○
Pregnancy Complication	●	●		●	○
Bone Loss	●	●	●		
Dental Decay	●	●			
Peridontal Disease	●	●	●	●	○
Implant Failure	●	●	●	●	○
Rheumatoid Arthritis		●			
Obesity		●			
Appendicitis		●			
Multiple Sclerosis		●			
Joint Replacement			●	●	
Cancer			●	●	○
Diabetes			●		
Oxidative Stress	●	●		●	
Intestinal Complications					○

Get regular cleanings and follow the advice of your dental professional. They are your best resource for learning to avoid oral systemic disease.

HOW CAN MY ORAL HEALTH PROFESSIONALS SUPPORT MY OPTIMAL HEALTH?

by Thomas Larkin, DDS

You have read how Oral health plays a more significant role in overall health than many realize. Inflammation and disease in the mouth can negatively impact the entire body, contributing to serious conditions. Bacterial, viral, and fungal pathogens linked to oral infections can lead to arterial disease (responsible for 50% of heart attacks and strokes), metabolic diseases like insulin resistance and Type 2 diabetes, cancer, dementia, high-risk pregnancies, and inflammatory arthritis.

Why isn't prevention more popular?

When I was in dental school, we were told that a vaccine or a magic pill would someday eliminate oral disease. For many dentists, this created a subliminal fear: what happens to your career if you're no longer needed?

This mindset, coupled with prevention's perceived lack of financial reward, has led many dentists to push it to the back of their minds. Instead, most have embraced what I call "transactional dentistry"—a repair-focused model. Patients visit to have a "hole" in their tooth patched or, in more advanced cases, undergo sophisticated procedures like CAD/CAM-milled crowns or $5,000 dental implants. While these technologies are impressive, they represent failures in prevention rather than successes in healthcare.

Dental disease causes extensive and avoidable damage to the mouth, despite being one of the easiest infections to treat. As I often remind patients: ***"A tooth removal is an amputation of a body part. Its replacement is a prosthesis. These are not healthcare successes—they are failures."***

Making Prevention Pay

Dental implants dominate today's trade journals. Over 3 million Americans have implants, and that number grows by 500,000 annually. The financial incentives are significant, with complete replacement cases sometimes costing up to $60,000. For dentists, the training, equipment, and infrastructure required for implants are costly but can yield extraordinary profits.

I recently heard of a dentist who placed $100,000 worth of implants in a single day. Compare that to a preventive-oriented dentist or physician who might work an entire year to earn a similar amount. This stark contrast highlights why prevention is often overlooked—it attracts purpose-driven professionals who prioritize patient health over financial gain.

A Profession Divided

A major trend reshaping dentistry is the rise of corporate Dental Service Organizations (DSOs). These corporations buy retiring dentists' practices, consolidate operations, and employ young dentists saddled with debt.

These transaction-based models prioritize cost, speed, and efficiency, catering to a disease/repair style of practice. One concerning trend is the presentation of large treatment plans with financing options during a patient's first visit—often before building trust or addressing the underlying causes of disease.

As I see it: *"Initial visits to the dentist should focus on biological disease assessment before moving toward restorative care."*

The Changing Insurance Paradigm

Insurance companies are ahead of the dental profession in recognizing the value of prevention. Research shows that healthier mouths lead to substantial medical cost savings. For example:

- Stroke patients: $5,168 annual savings
- Diabetes: $2,840
- Pregnancy: $2,433
- Heart disease: $1,090

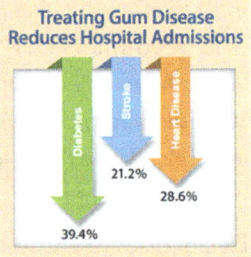

Image Source: Society of Teachers of Family Medicine

These findings demonstrate the financial and healthcare benefits of aggressive oral prevention. With 10,000 people reaching retirement age daily and wellness becoming a buzzword, insurance carriers are actively promoting preventive programs. This shift is driving renewed interest in prevention, as its true value becomes clear.

The Children of a Dentist

Children of dentists tend to have significantly lower rates of dental disease. Many never experience cavities, gum disease, implants, or dentures. Why? Here are three plausible reasons:

1. **Healthier biofilm**: Dental professionals likely maintain a healthier oral microbiome, reducing disease transmission to their children.
2. **Education**: Dentist-parents instill consistent oral hygiene habits and reinforce their importance.
3. **Access to the best practices**: Their families benefit from advanced preventive tools and techniques.

Notably, these advantages are not tied to financial privilege but rather to education and good information. Eliminating dental decay and gum disease is an achievable goal for anyone willing to adopt these practices.

As I often say: *"If it works for thousands of dentists and their families, it can work for you too."*

Proactive Oral Wellness

In 2016, I launched Proactive Oral Wellness—a comprehensive initiative aimed at educating both consumers and healthcare professionals about the vital connection between oral health and overall health. Over the years, I appeared on numerous podcasts and conducted countless webinars to spread awareness and drive meaningful conversations in this space.

In 2021, I began hosting live training events titled "The Future of Dental Hygiene." These events brought together a panel of experts specializing in cutting-edge technologies and innovative approaches to preventive dentistry. Through hands-on demonstrations and in-depth training, participants gained valuable insights into establishing a "Health-Centered Dental Practice." The overwhelming demand for these events, which consistently sell out well in advance, underscores the growing enthusiasm among providers to embrace this paradigm shift in dental care.

The Larkin Protocol

In 2020, I developed a precise training program for the early diagnosis and treatment of oral dysbiosis (infection), which became known as The Larkin Protocol. This groundbreaking protocol empowers dental professionals to address oral infections effectively, promoting optimal health outcomes for their patients.

Key Components of the Larkin Protocol

1. Advanced Diagnostics:

One of the key players in this oral-systemic connection is the bacteria in your mouth. There are both good and bad bacteria that inhabit the mouth, forming the "oral microbiome." The goal is to maintain barriers to invasion locally (gingivitis and periodontitis) and systemically (arterial injury), reduce the population of bad bacteria, and create an environment to promote good bacteria.

- Use of a microscope by the dental hygienist to display and educate patients about oral bacteria
- Saliva testing measures the presence and quantity of pathogenic bacteria.
- See the chart on page 72, which shows the relationship between high risk oral pathogens and systemic diseases
- Cone beam 3D CT scans are instrumental in detecting hidden infections or abscesses that may contribute to systemic inflammation. These issues, often asymptomatic, can go unnoticed during routine exams or standard X-rays. Old root canals, in particular, are common sites of chronic inflammation, which can be challenging to identify without the advanced imaging provided by CT scans. Such silent infections pose significant risks, as their first noticeable symptoms could manifest as severe events like a heart attack or stroke.
- Sleep screening, which can be seamlessly integrated into a dental exam, helps identify patients who may require a more comprehensive sleep study. Sleep disorders are a significant contributor to systemic inflammation.

2. Antimicrobial Therapy:

- Laser Therapy: Incorporates laser bacterial reduction (LBR) as a part of the cleaning protocol to target bad bacteria without harming beneficial microbes.
- Guided Biofilm Therapy: A new technology that identifies and gently removes risky biofilm with a warm medicated slurry of water and a medicated powder.
- The use of Ozonated water as an antimicrobial standard for all water lines used in the dental office.

3. pH Management: The protocol includes recommendations for pH-favorable rinses and Pre and Probiotic products to maintain an environment conducive to healthy bacterial balance.

4. Personalized Proactive Intervention Plans:
- Tailored to individual risk factors, these plans focus on daily oral hygiene practices, dietary adjustments, and professional follow-ups.
- Patients are educated about the link between oral pathogens and systemic conditions, empowering them to take proactive measures.

What Can I Do to Avoid Oral Health Issues?

1. Work with a Knowledgeable Dentist:
- Choose a dental professional who understands concerns beyond your teeth. Ensure your dentist has participated in continuing education about the oral-systemic connection, such as the Larkin Protocol.
- Look for a dentist with a Biological or Holistic designation.

2. Follow a Comprehensive Daily Home Care Routine:
- Brush and floss daily, use a water flosser, and incorporate pH-favorable mouth rinses.
- Consider Pre and Probiotics which assist in managing a healthy oral biofilm.

3. Get Regular Screenings and Tests:
- Saliva testing should be done at least once yearly to detect pathogenic bacteria.
- Cone beam CT scans are recommended for patients with prior cardiovascular events or elevated markers like myeloperoxidase (MPO).

4. Celebrate the long-term benefits:
- A healthy smile contributes to confidence and social well-being.
- Investing in preventive care can save tens of thousands of dollars in lifetime dental care expenditures
- Maintaining a healthy mouth has a profound effect on your overall health.

The Oral-Systemic Connection: A Pathway to Better Health

Maintaining oral health is a cornerstone of overall health. Programs like the Larkin Protocol provide a framework to reduce the burden of high-risk bacteria, protect barriers to invasiveness, and lower the risk of systemic diseases. By partnering with knowledgeable dental professionals and following evidence-based proactive intervention plans, you can optimize your overall health outcomes.

WHAT IS SLEEP APNEA? WHY SHOULD I TEST FOR IT?

Sleep apnea is characterized by repeated interruptions in breathing during sleep. This can occur when the muscles at the back of the throat fail to keep the airway open, causing an individual to struggle for air. Common symptoms of sleep apnea include loud snoring, daytime sleepiness, morning headaches, and difficulty concentrating. Sleep apnea can increase the risk of high blood pressure, heart disease, stroke, and other health problems. Contrary to common belief, thin people can suffer from sleep apnea and its consequences.

Why should I test for sleep apnea?

Sleep apnea has been found to contribute to:

- High blood pressure (proper treatment of sleep apnea can reduce or eliminate the need for blood pressure medications)
- Metabolic syndrome due to obesity (insulin resistance, prediabetes, Type 2 Diabetes)
- Atrial Fibrillation
- Dementia and other cognitive disorders
- Accidents and injuries
- Daytime fatigue/sleepiness

How do I test for sleep apnea?

Testing is now generally done at home with less expensive, user-friendly methods. In most cases, further testing is not necessary. Click here for a description of our favorite: EZ Sleep. However, if additional testing and treatment is needed, we refer you to sleep specialists, including dentists, who focus on sleep and airway disturbances.

What are the treatment options?

Choice of treatment for sleep apnea depends on its severity, underlying causes and patient preference. The goal of general treatment is to improve breathing during sleep and reduce symptoms and risk of complications.

Some common treatments include (but are not limited to):

- **Continuous Positive Airway Pressure (CPAP)**, which involves wearing a mask over your nose and mouth during sleep. CPAP opens your airway by delivering a steady stream of air under positive pressure.

- **Bi-level Positive Airway Pressure (BiPAP)**, which is similar to a CPAP but delivers less air while the user is exhaling. This is in contrast to CPAP, which delivers a constant stream of air, sometimes making it difficult for the user to exhale.

- **Mandibular advancement devices (MADs)**, also known as oral appliances, that can be worn in the mouth to help keep the airway open. They often accomplish this by bringing the jaw forward or holding the tongue in place.

- **Lifestyle changes** such as losing weight, quitting smoking, and avoiding alcohol before bedtime.

    While weight loss is helpful to treat sleep apnea (remove the root cause), often treatment of sleep apnea with CPAP or other measures enables weight loss. The cortisol and other stress consequences of sleep apnea make it harder to lose fat. It is a chicken/egg metaphor: Which comes first? In reality, obesity (even mild) and sleep apnea can be cause-and-effect for one another.

- **Nasal Decongestants** can sometimes be used to help open airways and improve breathing.

- **Positional therapy**, which involves using special devices or techniques to encourage sleeping on one's side.

- **Surgery**, which is usually a last resort, can be used to treat sleep apnea. In these rare cases, excess tissue is removed from the throat, or the jaw is repositioned to improve breathing during sleep.

- **Inspire**

Don't fear the diagnosis or the treatment of sleep apnea. Most who have been through it are grateful for better health and quality of life for themselves and their sleep partner.

WHAT IS LIPOPROTEIN A/LP(A)? DOES IT INCREASE RISK FOR HEART ATTACK & STROKE?

Lipoprotein A or Lp(a) is a subtype of LDL cholesterol. The BaleDoneen Method calls Lp(a) the "mass murderer" because elevated levels of Lp(a) triples your risk of heart attack and stroke. At the CureCenter, we call it the "worst" or "really bad" cholesterol. Think of it as "highly flammable" lipid.

Elevated Lp(a) affects around 30% of the population, yet it is not included in standard lipid testing. Why?

In the past, the test for Lp(a) was expensive. Today, it only costs about $10 and is becoming more common, yet still not routine. Change in practice tends to be slow, particularly in bureaucratic systems designed to keep revenue flowing through interventions. New drugs and associated revenue are on the horizon, potentially explaining a resurgence in interest.

What causes elevated Lp(a)?

Elevated Lp(a) is a genetically determined root cause with little impact from lifestyle or medications. Blame and warn your parents and siblings if it is high. Thank them if it is low. You are much more likely to have elevated Lp(a) if you have a family history of high Lp(a).

Why does elevated Lp(a) increase risk for heart attack and stroke?

Lp(a) is made of cholesterol, protein, and fat. Elevated levels (>75 mg/dl) increase the likelihood of development of atherosclerosis, leading to heart attack and stroke. Elevated Lp(a) also increases the risk of calcific aortic stenosis, a valve disease that can lead to heart failure. Finally, it accelerates blood clotting. When atherosclerotic plaque ruptures, a blood clot forms more rapidly to occlude blood flow leading to a stroke or heart attack.

When combined with high levels of inflammation, elevated Lp(a) fuels that inflammation in the artery wall and leads to the formation of plaque.

Lp(a) is not included in standard lipid panels ordered by most doctors. It should be.

While its effect is often lost in the statistics of large population studies, Lipoprotein (a) can be dangerous for the minority with significantly elevated levels. For this reason, everyone should have it measured once, especially if you have:

- Family members who have had a heart attack or stroke at an early age
- Premature vascular disease in the absence of other usual risk factors
- Familial hypercholesterolemia
- Family history of elevated Lp(a)

If your Lp(a) is tested and at a normal level, you will not need a repeat test. Your levels will not rise. However, if it is very high, you and your relatives should know, as they could be at high risk as well.

How are elevated levels of Lp(a) treated?

Niacin is the most effective supplement/drug to reduce levels of Lp(a). We have also witnessed response to Bergamot BPF, an effect we have not seen reported in the literature but have observed incidentally. In our experience Bergamot BPF has had a favorable effect that rivals or exceeds niacin in some cases, and it reduces insulin resistance, a highly prevalent root cause of atherosclerosis.

Lifestyle and statins tend to have very little effect on reducing high levels of Lp(a). They can, however reduce inflammation contribution to disease and cardiac events. Therefore, knowing about the increased risk from Lp(a) can motivate more proactive measures to control these other root causes more optimally.

Knowing about the presence of this "mass murderer" in your body will make healthy diet, exercise, and other risk reductions more imperative. Information is empowering. Become aware of Lp(a) - the "worst" or "really bad" cholesterol.

For further reading on Lipoprotein A, we recommend visiting BaleDoneen.com

WHAT ARE LDL AND HDL? HOW DO THEY AFFECT MY HEALTH?

Low-Density Lipoprotein (LDL) and High-Density Lipoprotein (HDL) are two types of lipoproteins (particles made of protein and fats/lipids) that transport cholesterol in the bloodstream.

LDL is often referred to as the "bad" cholesterol because it carries cholesterol from the liver to the cells and can build up in the blood vessels, increasing the risk of heart disease. However, this happens primarily to OXIDIZED LDL. LDL is oxidized by accumulating oxidative stress from toxin exposure.

HDL is considered the "good" cholesterol as it picks up excess cholesterol from the artery walls and takes it back to the liver to be removed from the body. But larger HDL is primarily responsible for this beneficial activity.

Maintaining a healthy balance of LDL and HDL cholesterol is important for overall health as high levels of LDL and low levels of HDL can increase the risk of heart disease and stroke, while high levels of HDL and low levels of LDL can help protect against heart disease. Regular exercise, a healthy diet, and avoiding smoking and excessive alcohol consumption can help maintain a healthy balance of LDL and HDL cholesterol levels.

However, there is more to LDL and HDL than a single reading. Small and large LDL and HDL affect cardiovascular health.

Large LDL is less risky and is commonly referred to as "buoyant" because it stays in circulation. This makes it less likely to penetrate the artery protective inner layer, literally bouncing off the wall like a beach ball. A preponderance of Large LDL is called a
Pattern A.

Small LDL is considered higher risk. It is more "dense," penetrating, and prone to get stuck in the wall to become fuel for inflammation which creates atherosclerotic plaque. A preponderance of Small LDL is called a Pattern B. It is associated with insulin resistance, the most common driver of arterial inflammation.

Large HDL removes cholesterol from the artery more efficiently than small HDL, transporting it to the liver for processing and removal.

To summarize, larger LDL and HDL particles reduce risk of arterial disease and events, while smaller LDL and HDL particles increase risk.

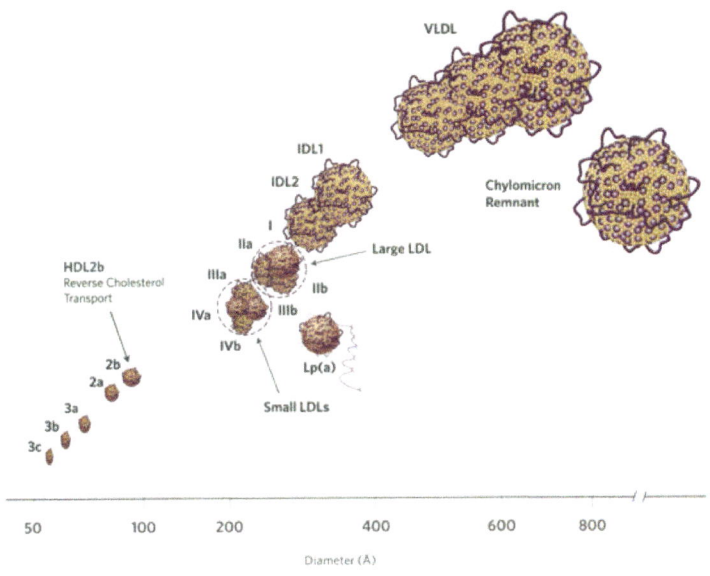

Image Source: Berkley Heart Lab

What causes smaller LDL and HDL in the body?

Smaller LDL and HDL particle size is commonly associated with insulin resistance (prediabetes, metabolic syndrome, Type 2 Diabetes), diets high in sugar and processed foods, smoking, and a sedentary lifestyle.

How can I increase the size of LDL and HDL in my body?

Lose fat (especially visceral fat), consume less sugar, starch and processed foods, including a significant amount of vegetables and fasting. Exercise (especially resistance training and increased muscle mass) is also a key driver of larger LDL and HDL production. Individuals with diabetes and prediabetes, should also work to improve control of these conditions, as they are also a factor in LDL and HDL size.

GENETIC TESTING: HOW DOES IT IMPACT ARTERIAL DISEASE?

Genetics play a significant role in whether you will have a heart attack or stroke. However, although we cannot yet alter our genes, we can "hack" them. Some genetic information can determine optimal treatment choices for you that may or may not be right for others (even those in the same family).

Lifestyle choices can change the way our genes are expressed (how the body uses information in our genes to create proteins and other molecules). This concept is called **epigenetics**.

Our genes are a blueprint for our bodies, but epigenetic changes can influence which genes are turned on or off. These changes can be passed down from one generation to the next, and can also be affected by our diet, exposure to toxins, and other factors. Studying epigenetics can help us understand how these changes occur, and how they may contribute to the development of diseases such as cancer and heart disease.

Genetic testing has become more affordable. Since it needs to be done only once, it is actually quite cost-effective even if insurance plans don't cover the costs. The sooner the information is know, the sooner changes in behavior or treatment can favorably impact the outcome.

Recommended genetic testing should emphasize tests for which there are meaningful remedies that can change the gene expression. Gene expression is the process by which our genes create proteins that perform different functions in our body, such as building and repairing tissues or fighting off infections.

Awareness of higher risk can provoke more proactive efforts on controllable factors. However, if you already have a disease, being "low risk" doesn't change your plan. You need to act on the disease to put it into remission.

On the other hand, those with high risk but no disease should not be exposed to the potential harms of treatment without benefit.

Genes determine how you metabolize medications. This can be important if you are on multiple medications that can interact with one another or require metabolism for elimination or activation. When inquiring about genetic testing, ask your doctor about these genes. Be wary of commercial panels of an array of genetic tests that can add more "noise" than "signal." 23 and Me offers little useful information for testing that really matters.

Knowing your genetics allows The CureCenter to individualize and personalize your care to lower your risk of having a heart attack or stroke. We offer limited genetic testing for all and encourage it especially for those who have had a heart attack, stroke, TIA, stent, bypass or signs of dementia to optimize treatment. For others, it enables the best possible choices to personalize your care.

Our rule: Order genetic tests that will determine a specific change in choices or prescriptions, especially when results are worse and trends are not favorable.

Genetic testing in low-risk individuals with no plan for lifestyle or treatment changes adds cost and noise with little signal.

What genetic tests are most helpful?

Haptoglobin genotype is very worthwhile, especially those with Type 2 Diabetes, insulin resistance, or prediabetes. Most of us fall into one of these categories!

The cost of this test has decreased significantly over the years. In 2018 the test cost about $400. Now, the cost is $99, a small price for precision in personalized treatment. Because it isn't offered by Quest or Cleveland Heart Lab, we use Boston Heart Diagnostics. We provide their kit to obtain the proper specimen as close to your home as possible at an affordable cost of $99 out of pocket. It is not covered by insurance, but this should not influence your opinion about whether it if "medically necessary."

How does haptoglobin genotype guide treatment?

The table below outlines the implications of knowing your haptoglobin genotype.

Result	Haptoglobin 1-1	Haptoglobin 1-2	Haptoglobin 2-2
Risk of Events (heart attack, stroke, etc.)	Normal	2x Normal Risk	5x Normal Risk
Gluten Effects	None	Moderate Inflammation	Severe Inflammation
Vitamin E Effects	Increased Risk of Events	Increased Risk of Events	Reduced Risk of Events
Results	Avoid Vitamin E	Avoid Vitamin E and Gluten	400 IU of Vitamin E Mixed with Tocopherols Daily; Avoid Gluten

Haptoglobin (Hp) 1-1 is the genotype at the lowest risk for vascular events such as heart attack or stroke. **Haptoglobin 1-2** doubles this risk (increases it by 200%). Both of these findings indicate that events are more likely to happen if an individual takes daily vitamin E supplements beyond what is contained in a multivitamin or diet.

Individuals with risk of macular degeneration may be taking supplements containing higher amounts of vitamin E. If your specialist is treating you for current macular degeneration, these supplements make sense. However, you should know that there is a trade off. Treating the risk of one condition may increase your risk of another. (See the table above for more information.)

Haptoglobin 2-2 genotype increases risk of vascular events by **500% (or 5x the baseline risk)**. Gluten should be avoided if this genotype is found, as it provokes a significant increase in inflammation, leading to a higher risk of events.

Individuals with the Haptoglobin 2-2 genotype should take a daily dose of 400 IU of Vitamin E mixed tocopherols to significantly reduce cardiovascular risk by 80%! The proof is greatest in those with Type 2 Diabetes, but most of us have the prediabetic curse that was a blessing when we ate like hunter gatherers.

What is the relevance of ApoE genotype?

We don't order ApoE routinely, but if you want it, we can order it. In select situations, it can help guide dietary choices, but are less relevant if insulin resistance and carbohydrate restriction is the more compelling opportunity. It often adds more "noise" than "signal."

The Apolipoprotein E (ApoE) genotype is a genetic factor that plays a significant role in various aspects of human health, particularly in relation to lipid metabolism and the risk of developing certain diseases. The ApoE gene encodes a protein that is involved in the transport and metabolism of lipids, including cholesterol, in the body. There are three common variants or alleles of the ApoE gene: ApoE2, ApoE3, and ApoE4.

The relevance of ApoE genotype lies in its association with several health conditions, including:

- **Alzheimer's/Dementia**: The ApoE4 allele is the strongest known genetic risk factor for late-onset Alzheimer's disease (AD). Individuals who inherit one copy of the ApoE4 allele from either parent have an increased risk of developing AD, while those who inherit two copies have an even higher risk. But if you are really interested in reducing your risk of dementia, read *Healthy Heart Healthy Brain* by Bale and Doneen and *The End of Alzheimer's* by Dale Bredesen.

- **Cardiovascular Disease**: The ApoE genotype is also linked to the risk of developing cardiovascular diseases such as coronary artery disease and stroke. ApoE4 carriers have been found to have higher levels of LDL cholesterol (often referred to as "bad" cholesterol) and an increased susceptibility to atherosclerosis, a condition characterized by the buildup of plaque in the arteries.
- **Lipid metabolism**: The ApoE genotype influences how the body metabolizes lipids. ApoE2 is associated with lower levels of cholesterol and a reduced risk of cardiovascular disease, while ApoE4 is associated with higher cholesterol levels and an increased risk.
- **Traumatic brain injury (TBI)**: Research suggests that the ApoE4 allele may be associated with an increased risk of poorer outcomes following TBI, including a higher likelihood of developing neurodegenerative disorders later in life.

It's important to note that while the ApoE genotype can provide insights into an individual's predisposition to certain conditions, it does not determine with certainty whether someone will develop these diseases. Other genetic and environmental factors generally play a more compelling modifiable role, and individual health outcomes are complex and multifactorial. Genetic testing and counseling can help individuals understand their ApoE genotype and its implications, but it's always best to consult with a healthcare professional for personalized advice and interpretation of genetic information.

What is the relevance of the KIF6 genotype?

We rarely order the KIF6 genotype. Our preference for rosuvastatin makes it largely irrelevant to guide treatment. If you insist on using atorvastatin, pravastatin or simvastatin, I suggest verifying this is wise based on KIF6 predicting benefit.

The KIF6 (kinesin-like protein 6) genotype refers to a specific genetic variation in the KIF6 gene. This gene has been studied in relation to cardiovascular health and response to certain medications. However, it is important to note that the current understanding of the relevance of KIF6 genotype is limited, and more research is needed to fully understand its implications.

The KIF6 gene variant in question is known as KIF6 719Arg. It has been associated with an increased risk of coronary artery disease (CAD) and heart attacks in some studies. Individuals who carry this genetic variant may have a higher likelihood of developing these cardiovascular conditions compared to those without the variant.

The KIF6 gene has also been investigated in the context of statin medications, which are commonly prescribed to lower cholesterol levels, suppress arterial inflammation and reduce the risk of cardiovascular events. Some studies have suggested that individuals with the KIF6 719Arg variant may experience a greater reduction in cardiovascular events when treated with statins compared to those without the variant. However, these findings have not been consistently replicated across all studies.

There is evidence that those with the KIF6 719Arg variant get more benefit from atorvastatin and pravastatin than those not carrying that variant. We prefer rosuvastatin as effective despite genetic variation and less prone to exacerbate insulin resistance/diabetes or cross the blood/brain barrier affecting cognition. Most of our patients take 5 mg 3 days weekly or less with benefit documented with blood and ultrasound inflammation measures.

It's important to understand that genetic factors, including the KIF6 genotype, are just one piece of the puzzle when it comes to cardiovascular health. Other factors such as lifestyle choices (e.g., diet, exercise), family history, and other genetic variations collectively contribute to an individual's risk for developing cardiovascular conditions.

Overall, while the KIF6 genotype has shown some associations with cardiovascular health and response to statin therapy, its clinical utility is still being explored, and further research is needed to determine its exact relevance and potential implications in healthcare practice.

9p21 Genotype is the Heart Attack Gene. It is the one to beat, as the title of Dr. Bale and Dr. Doneen's book suggests. However, there is no specific treatment for this gene. Its presence could motivate someone sitting on the fence about some treatments, but for the most part, we rarely order it since our program is based upon measurable disease, not risk.

MTHFR (Methyl tetra hydrofolate reductase) gene variants can increase the methylated folic acid need to maintain safe levels of homocysteine. Homocysteine elevation raises incidence of stroke, heart attack, neuropathy, kidney failure and blood clotting.

COVID-19: WHAT SHOULD I KNOW? WHAT SHOULD I DO?

Be Empowered. Be Safe. Be Resilient and Resistant to COVID (and other threats) to your health and well being.

At the CureCenter, we believe that working to **reverse and cure chronic disease** not only improves overall health, but also **protects you** from infection and other consequences of viruses such as Covid-19. In our experience, resilience and general immunity that accompanies good health is more effective (and safer) than any available vaccine.

There is abundant evidence early treatment protocols, regardless of vaccination choices, can reduce severity of illness, hospitalization, and death from Covid-19. This includes optimized vitamin D levels to 50+ mg/dl.

The CDC has admitted that chronic disease severely increases risk of serious illness or death from Covid-19. The large majority of Covid deaths occur in those with diabetes, arterial disease, obesity, and hypertension. Almost nobody with a vitamin D3 level above 50 died from COVID. Levels below 20 were typical of those who died.

So why are most public health officials not pointing out this obvious opportunity to improve health, reduce mortality overall? It is a combination of complacency and complicity with Big Food, Big Pharma and the rest of the medical industrial complex that is making more profit from vaccines and non-generic therapeutics than from prevention and effective early treatment.

Should I get the Covid-19 vaccine and/or boosters?

Our advice: Think for yourself, consider your circumstances, and then decide.

The older and sicker you are, the more the vaccines make some sense. The healthier and younger you are, consider the risk as well as the purported benefit. Seek information from a variety of sources. Debate, not censorship or suppression of information, is the hallmark of science. "Science" is a process, not a person or specific recommendation or consensus opinion, no matter the source, their seniority or their position of authority.

Covid exposure risk will wax and wane. New variants will emerge. "Vaccines" have not been as effective or safe as originally hoped/hyped. These "vaccines" have made the most sense for highly vulnerable populations but make little, if any, sense for children and young healthy adults. It is the antithesis of safety to recommend these insufficiently (and some sources suggest fraudulently) tested injections in pregnancy for the safety of mother and baby. There have been so many examples of public health recommendations that violate basic time proven principles, especially informed consent and do no harm.

Their main benefit thus far has been reduction in hospitalization and death from Covid-19 in high risk individuals. However, they do not prevent infection or spread. Since this is the usual expectation of vaccines, one would logically ask if they are, in fact, "vaccines" at all.

At this point in time, there is no way to know enough about the long term safety or efficacy of the mRNA "vaccines." They were rushed into use far more rapidly than other approved vaccines without usual testing or trials. There is also no evidence that immunity from vaccines is superior to immunity from infection with Covid-19. In fact, the opposite is more likely to be true.

At the CureCenter, we promote our patients taking an active role in their own health. We suggest that you seek information less biased by commercial interest and think logically and with less emotion based on what you find. Consider the motivation and bias in the sources you seek out. What are the selling? It is also always a good idea to "follow the money."

If you are convinced of the benefit of the mRNA vaccines, get vaccinated. Advocate for protection for your community, but please do not demand that others follow your lead if they come to an opposite conclusion. Mandates, vaccine passports, and coercion are authoritarian measures that increase resistance and rarely change minds. All individuals should be free to choose and accept the consequences of their own choices. You get a vaccination to protect yourself, not others. If you have been vaccinated with a safe and effective product, someone who has not consented to the same is not a threat. If it isn't safe and effective, why would anyone trust the benefit of demanding that someone else act to protect us?

A few additional things to consider:

- Covid-19 proves fatal mainly to those with heart disease and diabetes. There is also evidence that the mRNA vaccines exacerbate arterial endothelial inflammation. Both of these can be prevented, reversed, and even put into remission. Control of preexisting arterial inflammation makes inflammation induced by spike protein less severe and a lesser threat.

- Hyperlipidemia is one of the few comorbidities that was associated with REDUCED risk of death. Why?

Could it be that the common treatment for hyperlipidemia (statins and other antiinflammatory strategies) actually mitigated the inflammation in COVID and saved lives?

- If you get spike protein inflammation either from infection or injection, it won't be as serious if your arteries and metabolism are already healthy.

    Ignorance may be bliss, but it's a terrible choice. Be empowered by understanding and improving your arterial age and metabolic health.

It's better to address underlying root causes of issues related to Covid death than to jump directly to an unproven vaccine.

How can I most effectively prevent serious illness or death from Covid-19?

The best way to prevent serious illness or death from any infection or disease, including Covid-19, is to be resilient, treat it early and avoid its source. This involves lifestyle changes such as healthy diet and exercise, proper sleep, reduced stress, and supplements and/or medication when appropriate.

If you or a loved one needs to reverse known or suspected chronic disease, such as arterial disease or Type 2 Diabetes, we suggest you visit **theCureCenter.life** to schedule a quick and painless 5-minute CureScreen carotid ultrasound. We will use this to determine your threat and put you on the best CurePlan for prevention of events by stopping progression.

Don't allow fear of exposure to Covid-19 keep you from necessary care for other conditions, including support for your mental and oral health.

CONCLUSION

I hope you agree that the time invested in this concise overview has proven valuable. For those who want more general and detailed information, there are many resources at **theCureCenter.life**.

Buckminster Fuller said: "You never change things by fighting the existing reality. To change something, build a new model that makes the existing model obsolete."

When you are ready to get started, visit our website and schedule a Discovery Zoom Call to find the best way to start your CurePlan journey.

For those loved ones in your life who need this message, please share this booklet with them.

Thank you for reading my message.

Craig Backs MD

Made in the USA
Monee, IL
06 March 2025